food for life

First published by Jane Curry Publishing
(Wentworth Concepts Pty Ltd T/A) 2006
220a Glenmore Road, Paddington, NSW 2021
www.janecurrypublishing.com.au

Text © Petrea King 2006

Design © Jane Curry Publishing 2006

Photography © Andre Martin 2006

National Library of Australia
cataloguing-in-publication data:

Petrea King, 1951- .

Food for life : recipes to enhance life.

Includes index.

ISBN 1 920727 25 6.

1. Cookery (Natural foods). I. Petrea King Quest for Life Centre.

II. Title.

641.563

Photography: Andre Martin
Food editor and stylist: Sally Parker
Home economist: Julie Ballard
Assistants: Dianne Stynes and Adam Trevanion
Typeset in Vista Sans
Printed in Singapore by Imago Productions

food for life

Petrea King
Quest for Life Centre

Recipes compiled by Sally Parker

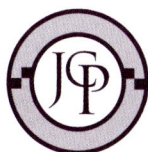

Jane Curry Publishing

acknowledgments

This collection of recipes was first promised in my book, *Quest for Life*, almost fifteen years ago. Without the determination and hard work of Sally Parker that promise would have remained unrealised. Sally very generously donated her time and expertise to gather and formulate these recipes as well as testing and styling them for photography. Thank you Sally for your patience and relentless good humour as we tweaked, edited and contributed more ideas to the finished product.

The photographer, Andre Martin, has captured the visual appeal of these dishes and John Dermer's pottery (Kirby's Flat Pottery, Yackandandah, Victoria) provides perfect plates and platters for the food's presentation. Thanks also to Dinosaur Designs and T2.

Maureen Williams also deserves special thanks for her contributions and willingness to co-ordinate the fermentation of the ingredients within these pages. Her persistence and encouragement helped me to complete this project.

Elspeth Menzies at Jane Curry Publishing made excellent suggestions as she too is passionate about healthy foods that sustain and improve wellbeing.

My gratitude goes to Doug Hughes, the chef at the Petrea King Quest for Life Centre, who infuses his creations with love and care and for whom no diet is too difficult to accommodate. Doug's delicious meals nourish the spirit and psyche of our guests as well as their physical bodies.

Petrea King
Founder, Petrea King Quest for Life Centre

All royalties from the sale of this book will go to the Quest for Life Foundation.

contents

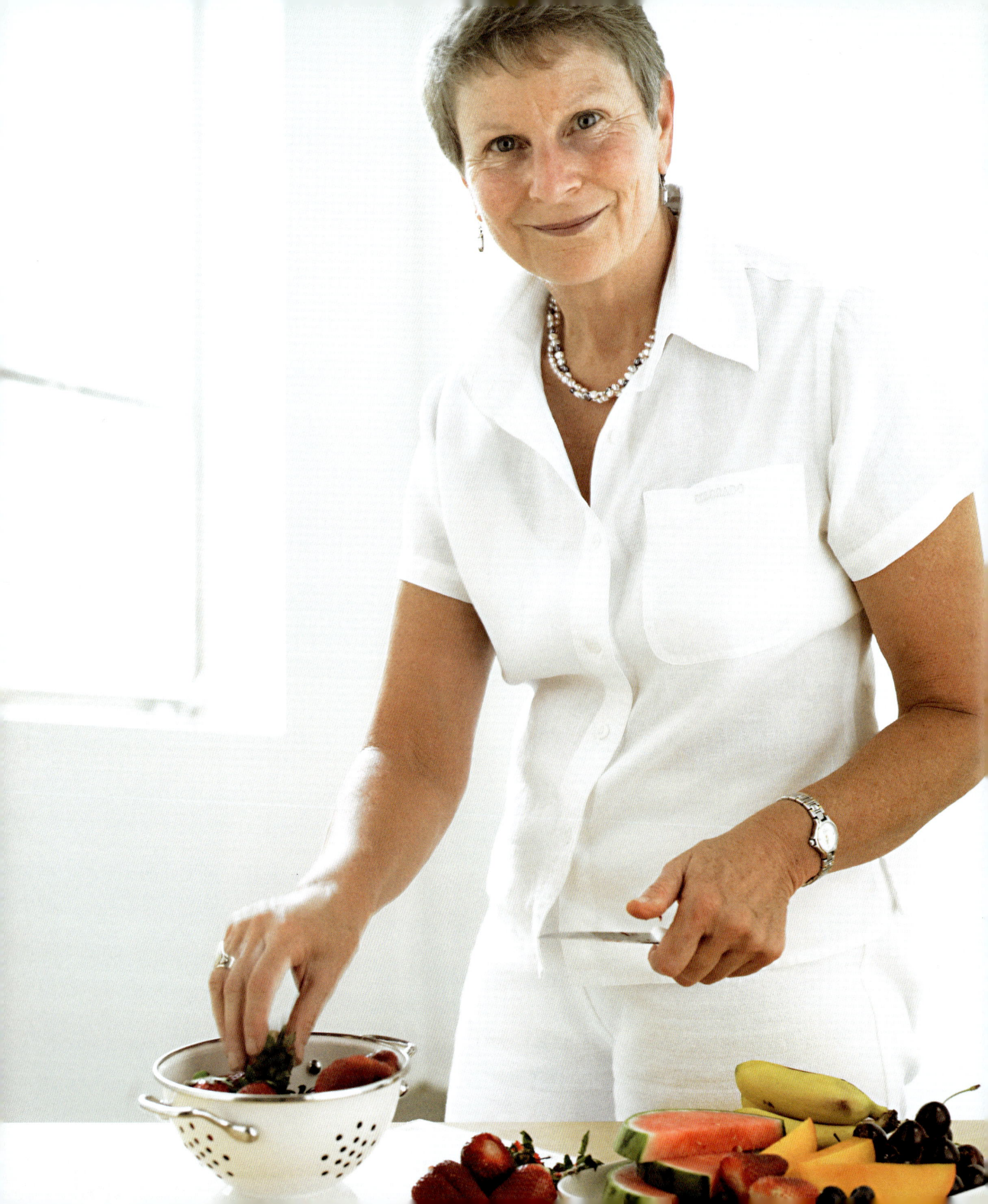

introduction

'Can I have the recipe?'
'How does Doug make vegetables taste so delicious?'
'What's the special ingredient?'
'If I could eat food like this for the rest of my life, I'd be happy and healthy!'

SINCE THE OPENING of the Quest for Life Centre in 1998 these and a myriad of other questions have been asked of our chef Doug Hughes and his staff.

The participants who attend residential programs at the Centre are often facing significant challenges in their lives. Many of our guests are living with life-threatening illnesses or neurological disorders and have special dietary requirements. Other people come to make meaning of grief, depression, trauma or anxiety or to regain a sense of identity after some significant loss. Some people are at a crossroad in their life and attend programs to deepen their self-understanding and clarify their values and direction. Regardless of why people come to the Quest for Life Centre, mealtimes are eagerly anticipated and are always a source of pleasure.

Though the dietary needs of our guests may differ widely, the philosophy of natural, seasonal and whole foods underpins every dish. The serving of fresh, healthy, seasonal food is integral to the Centre's programs and it is gratifying to see the physical improvement in our guests' health over the space of a few days — good food really does nourish the spirit as well as the body.

So many of our guests have wanted to take Doug home with them at the end of their program! So instead of him telling us 'it's a dash of this and a handful of that', we have finally extracted written recipes from Doug and, along with a few other favourites, we are delighted to bring you *Food for Life*.

More than anything, these recipes are simply wholesome and delicious and will be enjoyed by the entire family. Throughout the book there are practical tips to incorporate into every lifestyle as well as some delicious recipes for people on restrictive diets. However, I would encourage you to listen to your intuition and choose a diet that feels right for you.

The following collection of recipes will have your mouth watering and I wish you health, healing and ever increasing vitality as you explore the wonderful world of Food for Life.

As a naturopath and herbalist for more than thirty years I have witnessed the profound benefits of a healthy, life-enhancing diet both in myself and in the more than 60,000 people who have attended our residential programs or sought counselling with me. A positive attitude combined with meditation, appropriate nutrition and a healthy lifestyle can lead to miracles.

My first interest in addressing my own dietary needs came about when I was crippled with arthritis in my early twenties after more than a dozen major surgeries to my legs during my teens. I was often reduced to relying on crutches and my orthopaedic surgeons' prognosis was that I would be crippled for life and unable to walk beyond my thirties. I tried many extreme 'naturopathic' diets and my experience has included extensive fasting both on water and juices and mono-diets and I was a strict vegan for fifteen years.

In my thirties I was diagnosed with acute myeloid leukaemia and again, diet played an important role in my recovery and my understanding of food and its role in our health. Now I listen to my body and eat what feels right for me. It's taken a lot of study and experimentation to finally have faith in my own common sense!

The following collection of recipes will have your mouth watering and I wish you health, healing and ever increasing vitality as you explore the wonderful world of food for life.

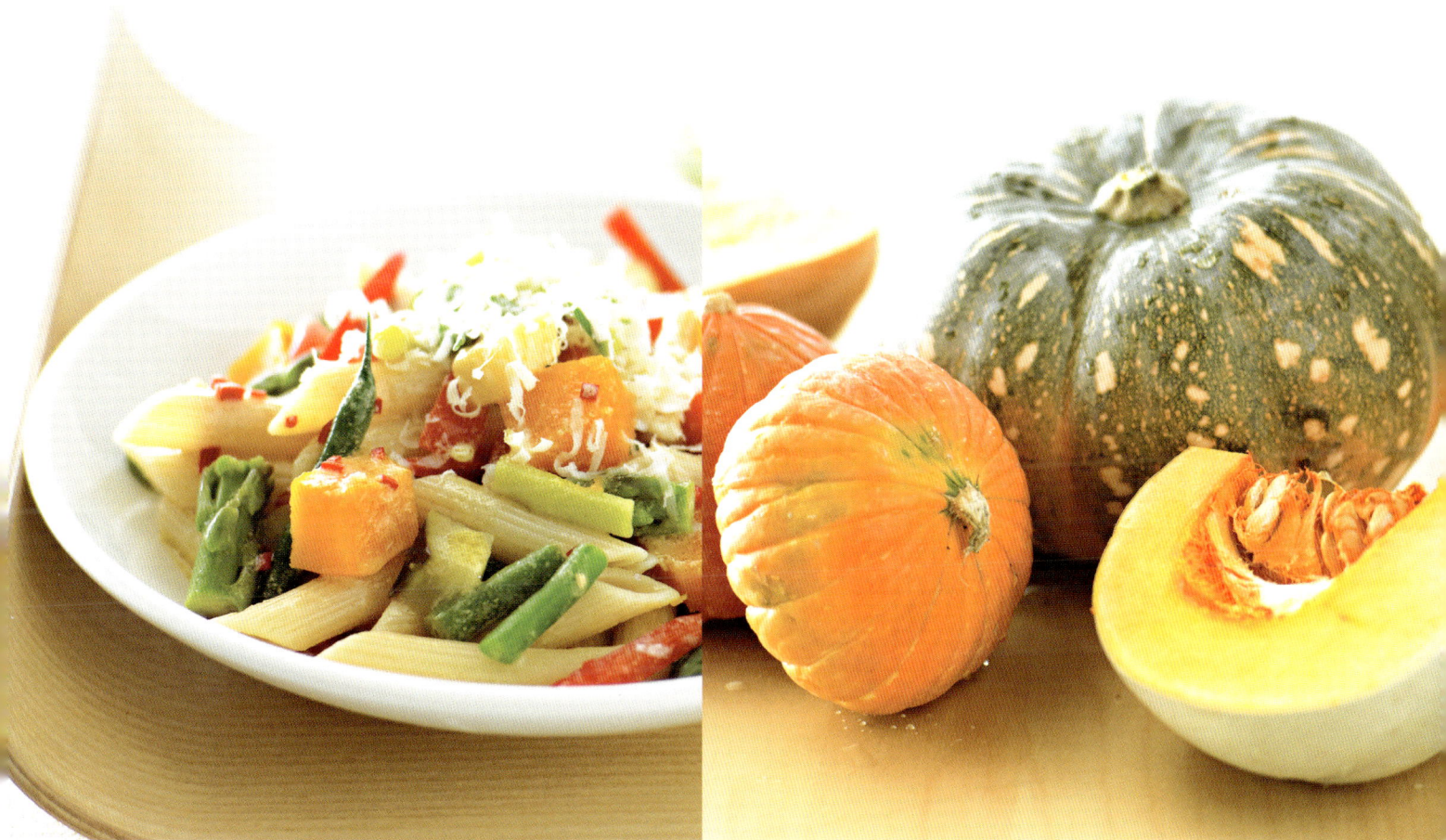

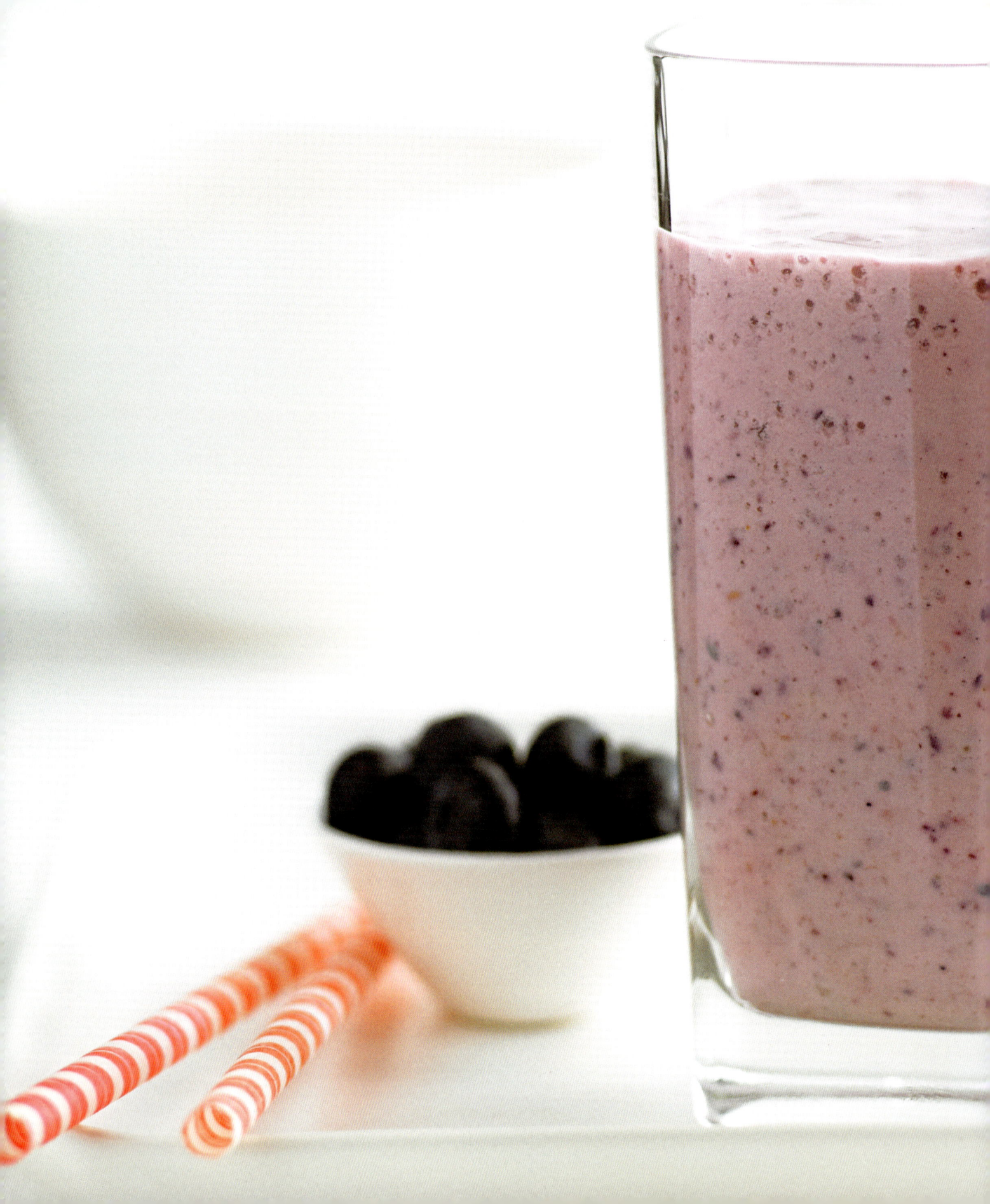

Juices,
Smoothies
& Drinks

juices, smoothies & drinks

Juices and smoothies are an excellent source of nutrients and are easy to both consume and digest. A freshly made juice is one of the best starts to any day.

OUR BODIES ARE made up of 85 per cent water and drinking juices, in addition to water, keeps us well hydrated. They also assist the body in flushing out toxins, and help our organs to function efficiently. Fruit juices are excellent internal cleansers and vegetable juices, which also nourish and cleanse, are generally gentler in their action.

Freshly made vegetable juices are an excellent addition to every diet, providing a fantastic array of vital vitamins, enzymes, antioxidants, minerals and trace elements.

Our bodies can quickly absorb the nutrients in fruit and vegetable juices which accelerates their cleansing potential and for people with low energy levels, who are feeling unwell or recovering from illness, vegetable juices can work wonders. Juices should always be freshly prepared and drunk immediately as storing them allows vital enzymes, antioxidants and vitamins to oxidise.

Except for the obvious fruits like mango, papaya, mandarins, pineapples, grapefruit, oranges and bananas, you don't need to peel fruits and vegetables if they are washed or scrubbed well. Juiced lemons and limes add a delicious tang to juices. And some people like to dilute their juices with a little water. To help digestion, it is best to drink juices at least 15 minutes before a meal or one and a half hours after. This allows the food in your stomach to be mixed effectively with gastric enzymes and hydrochloric acid rather than be diluted with juice or water.

Smoothies are deliciously nourishing and are great if you don't feel like eating, are underweight or having digestive problems. Smoothies are also great for hungry children and teenagers who can't manage to chew anything at breakfast! Coconut milk is a nutritious and delicious alternative to cow's milk — keep some tins in the pantry so you always have it on hand to include in smoothies, soups and other dishes.

We also have some great alternatives to the perennial coffee and tea. Reducing caffeine will reward you with better sleep and more consistent energy.

We serve many different delicious and healthy juices, smoothies and drinks at the Quest for Life Centre — here are some of our favourites.

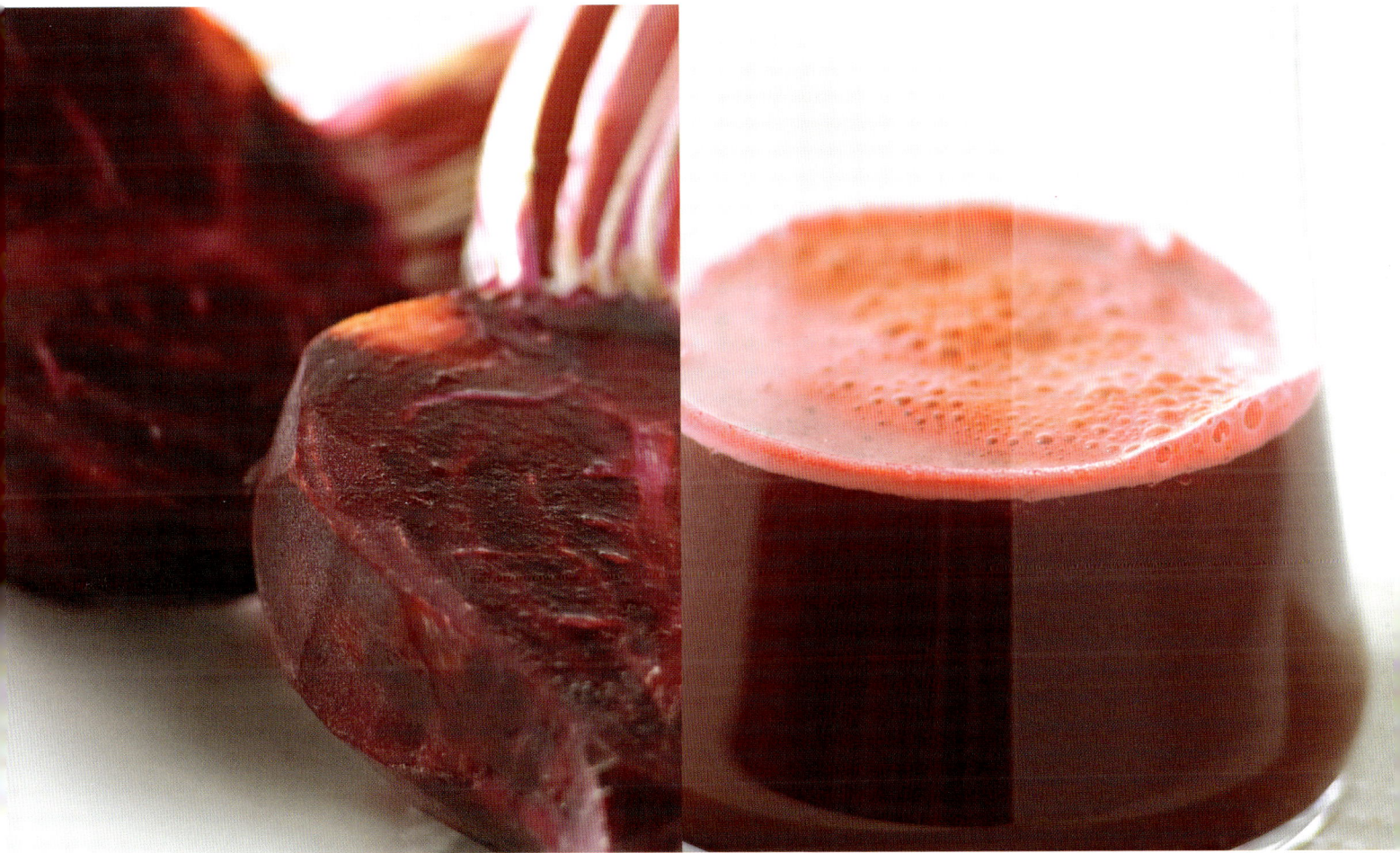

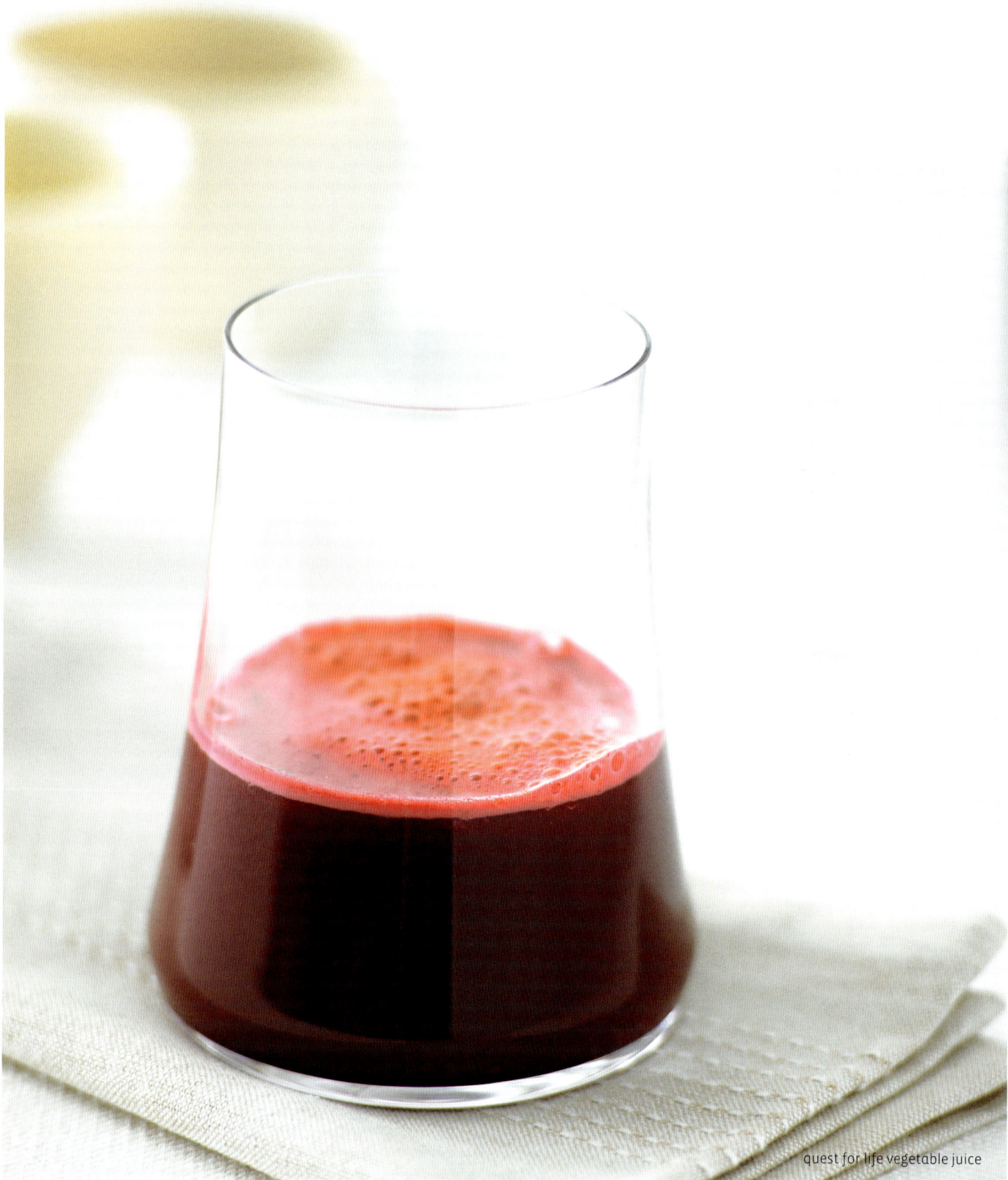

quest for life vegetable juice

Carrots are rich in beta carotene and beetroot stimulates liver function and is a powerful blood cleanser and builder. You might like to add a small knob of ginger, a clove of garlic or a whole lime to this recipe. The quantity the recipe will make depends on the juiciness and size of the carrots. The proportions of this juice should be around 85 per cent carrot juice, 10 per cent beetroot juice and 5 per cent green juice.

4 carrots, scrubbed, 1^1/$_2$ cm cut off the top
1 small beetroot, scrubbed, topped and tailed
1 stick celery or 1 large spinach leaf or dark green lettuce
    leaf or ^{1}/$_2$ cup parsley leaves

Chop the carrots and beetroot into pieces suitable to go through a juicer. Put the green vegetable through before the beetroot and carrot. If using parsley, wrap in a lettuce leaf to push through the juicer. Drink within 5 minutes to maximise the nutritional benefits. Makes 1 glass.

carrot, celery and pineapple juice

The pineapple in this juice makes it sweeter and for some, more palatable.

5 carrots, scrubbed, 1^1/$_2$ cm cut off the top
3 sticks celery, washed
1 cup chopped pineapple

Process the carrot, celery and pineapple through a juicer, and drink immediately. Makes 2 glasses.

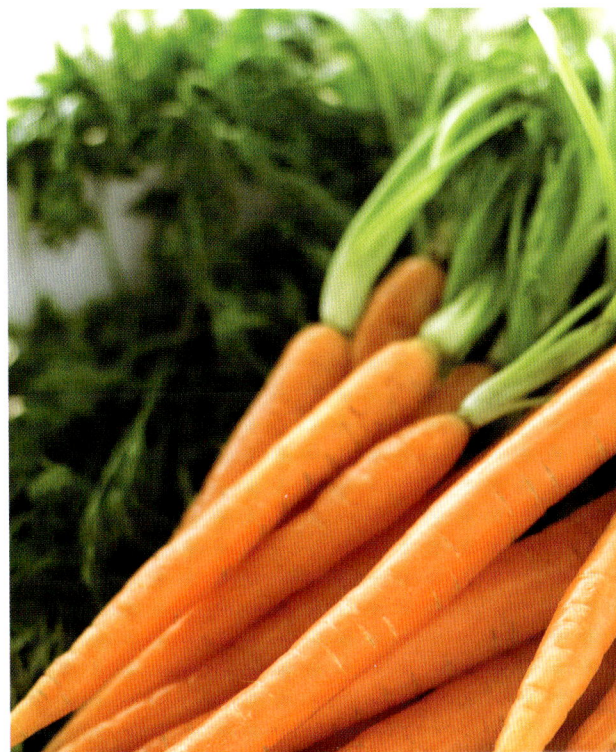

beetroot, cucumber and carrot juice

This juice is a variation on the Quest for Life vegetable juice adding cucumber for a clean, fresh taste.

4 carrots, scrubbed, 1 ^{1}/$_2$ cm cut off the top
1 medium beetroot, scrubbed, topped and tailed
1 Lebanese cucumber or ^{1}/$_3$ telegraph cucumber, washed
^{1}/$_2$ cup parsley leaves

Chop the vegetables into pieces suitable to go through a juicer, and push through a juicer along with the parsley. Drink immediately. Makes 2 glasses.

beetroot blend

Beetroot is a great blood builder, ginger promotes digestion and celery is an excellent diuretic. This blend gets the body's juices flowing and is delicious as well.

2 large beetroots, scrubbed, topped and tailed
5 sticks celery with leaves on, washed
2 pears, cored and quartered
3cm piece ginger

Juice together and serve immediately. Makes 2 glasses.

watercress cooler

Cucumber is an excellent internal cleanser and watercress is rich in calcium, chlorophyll and antioxidants. The green apples add colour, a tart sweetness and nutrition.

2 small Lebanese cucumbers or 1 telegraph cucumber
3 cups watercress
4 green apples, washed, quartered and unpeeled

Juice the cucumber first, then the watercress and finish off with the apple. You can feel this recipe doing you good! Makes 2 glasses.

super green juice

This juice often alleviates a headache and fixes constipation!

2 large carrots, scrubbed, $1^{1}/_{2}$ cm cut off the top
dozen leaves English spinach
4 sticks celery with leaves on, washed
2 sticks silver beet, washed

Juice everything together leaving the carrots until last and drink immediately. Makes 1 glass.

melon, pineapple and ginger juice

Fresh ginger is delicious and adds spiciness to this juice. It's best to push soft fruits through a juicer more slowly to extract the maximum amount of juice. You can use watermelon, honeydew or rockmelon. Adding a whole lime makes it wonderfully refreshing.

1 cup chopped melon
1 cup chopped pineapple
3cm piece ginger

Process the melon, pineapple and ginger through a juicer into a glass and drink immediately. Makes 1 glass.

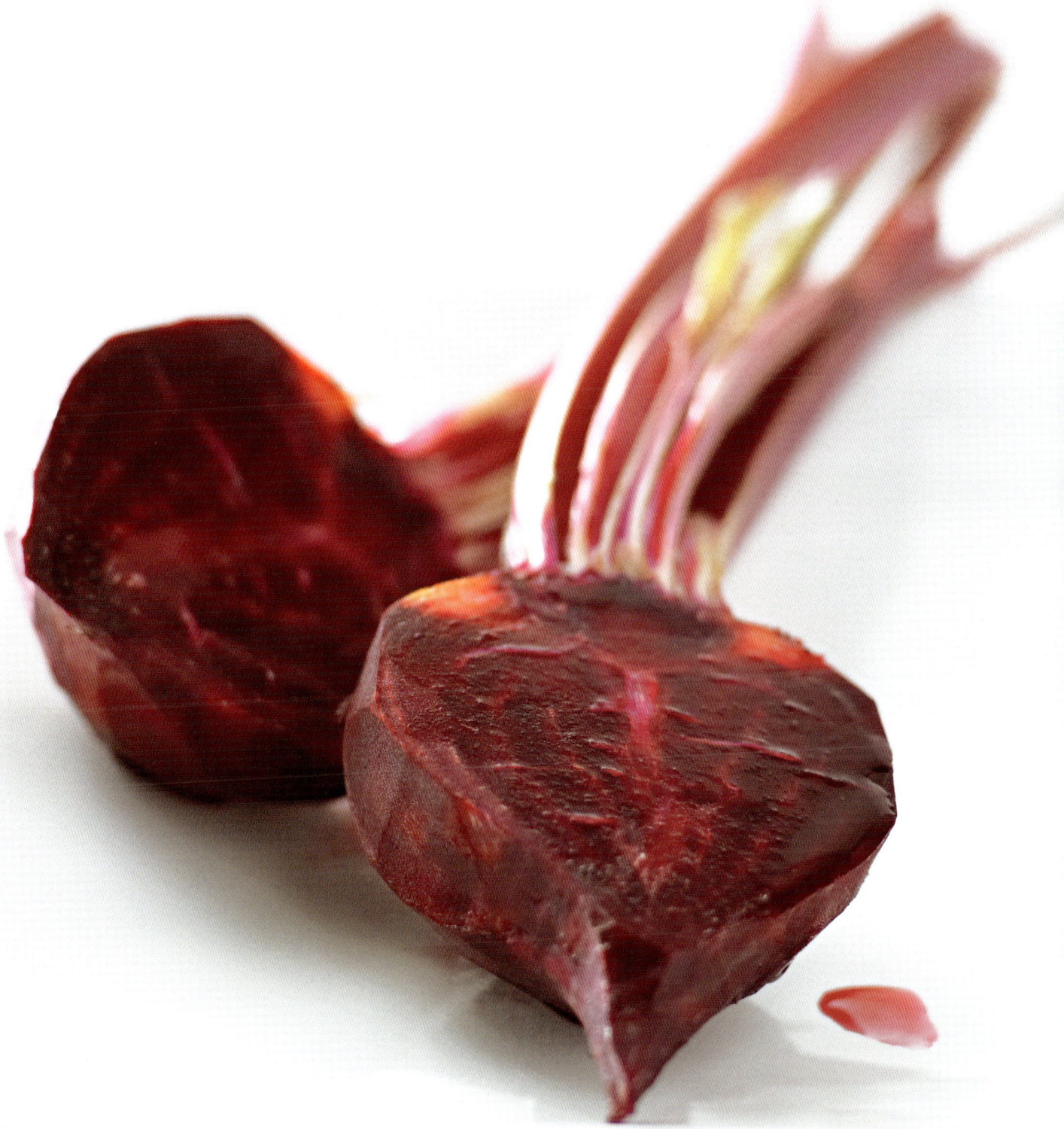

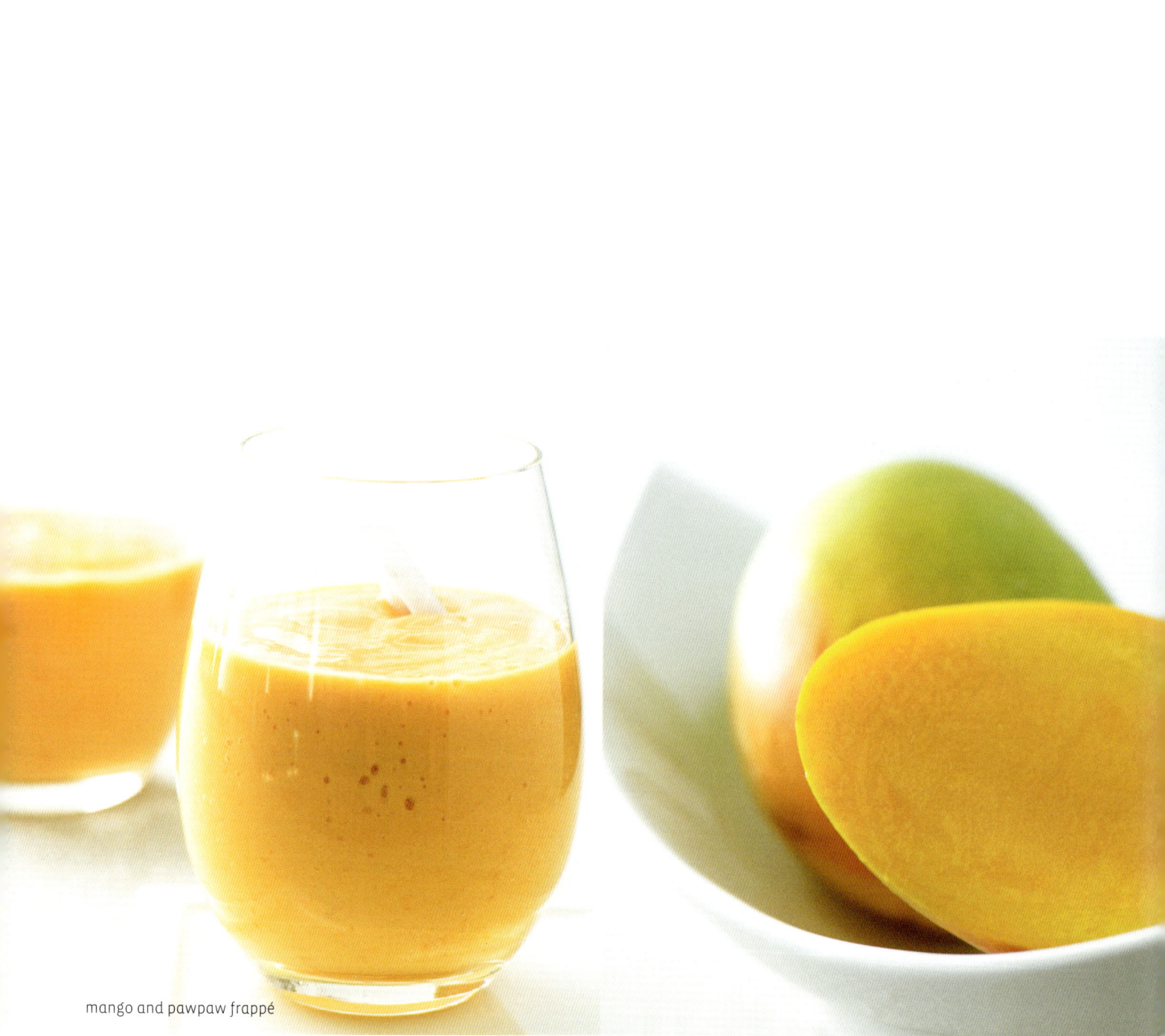

mango and pawpaw frappé

ruby delight

This delicious and refreshing juice will quench your thirst on the hottest day.

3 large peaches, pitted and quartered
2 punnets strawberries, hulled
2 ruby grapefruits, peeled
1/2 cup fresh mint leaves

Juice the peaches, strawberries and then the mint leaves before the grapefruit to extract the full flavour. Decorate with a mint leaf or two. Makes 2 glasses.

mango and pawpaw frappé

Celebrate summer and the prolific quantities of mangoes with this refreshing frappé.

3 mangoes, peeled and flesh chopped
1 cup chopped paw paw
1 lime, juiced
1/2 cup sparkling mineral water
1/2 cup plain yoghurt
1/2 cup ice cubes or crushed ice

Place all the ingredients in a food processor or blender and blend until smooth. Pour into 2 glasses and serve immediately.

Pile blueberries, raspberries, blackberries and green grapes into tall frosted glasses with a dollop of yoghurt and a decorative mint leaf.

fruit frappé

In the summer months you might like to keep a couple of glasses in the fridge to serve this delicious frappé.

1/2 cup chopped fresh pineapple
1 pear, cored and quartered
1 banana, chopped
1/2 cup raspberries, frozen or fresh
1 cup fresh orange or ruby grapefruit juice
1 tablespoon fresh mint leaves
6 ice cubes

Place the chopped pineapple, pear, banana, raspberries and orange juice or ruby grapefruit juice in a blender. Add the ice cubes and blend until thick and smooth. Pour into 2 large chilled glasses and garnish with mint leaves.

banana smoothie

A banana smoothie provides excellent and delicious nourishment for someone who's feeling a little frail, is underweight or having digestive problems. It's also great for those who just love smoothies! This recipe can be safely stored in the fridge for a day.

1 large banana
1 1/2 cups milk (cow, oat, brown rice or coconut)
2 tablespoons plain yoghurt
1 egg (optional)
pinch of cinnamon
1 teaspoon honey (optional)

Place all the ingredients in a blender or food processor and blend until smooth. Pour into a glass and serve.
Makes 2 glasses.

pear and coconut smoothie

The addition of coconut cream and milk to a smoothie is an easy way to increase healthy protein. Make sure the pears you use are ripe and juicy.

4 ripe pears, cored and quartered
400ml can coconut milk
2 tablespoons coconut cream
1/2 cup plain yoghurt
1/2 cup milk (cow, oat or brown rice)

Place all the ingredients into a blender or food processor and blend until smooth. Pour into 2 glasses and drink immediately.

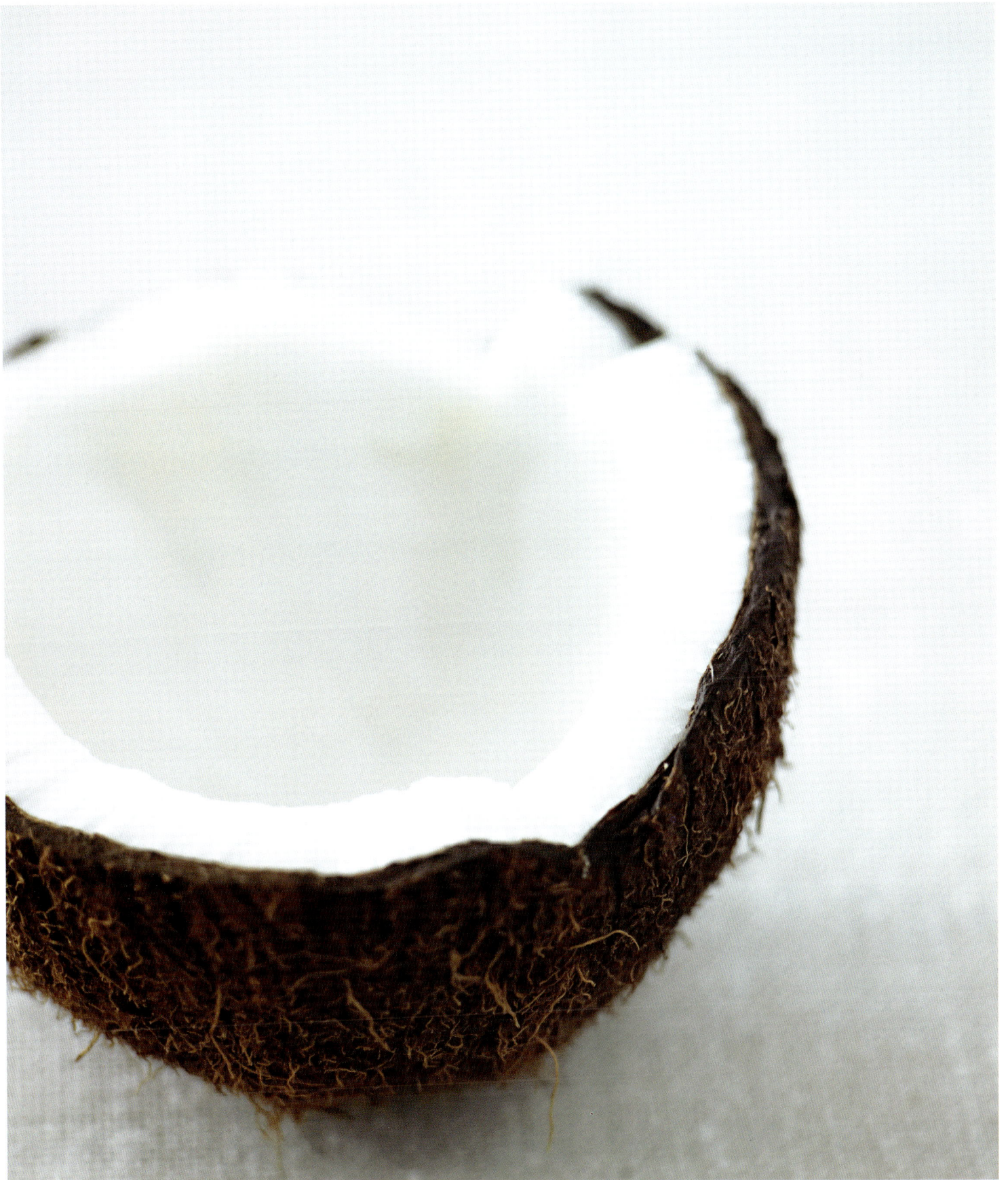

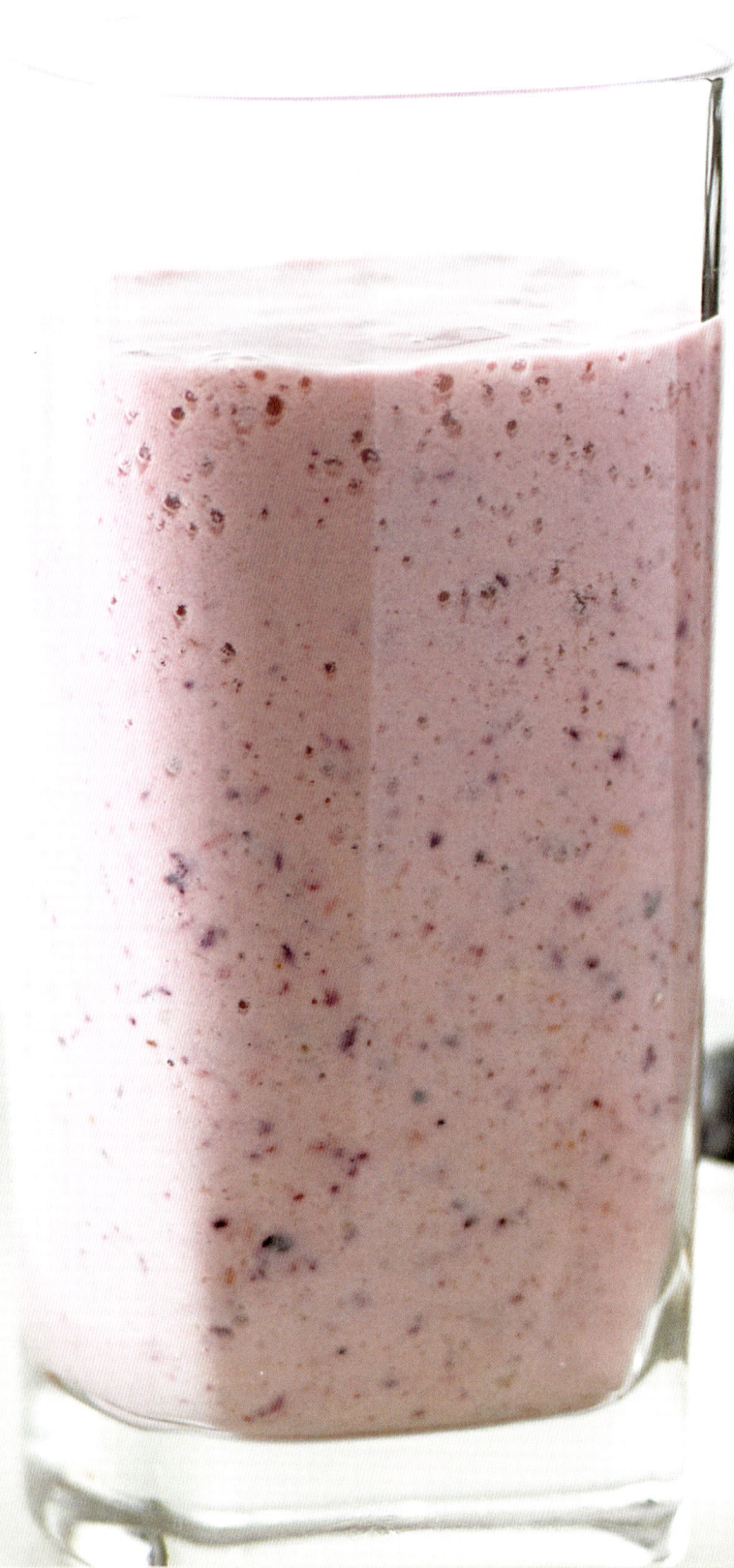

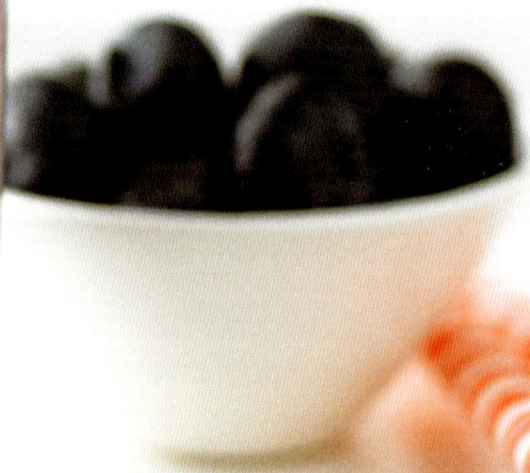

berry smoothie

berry smoothie

This is a fabulous smoothie, especially for hungry children or teenagers. A spoonful or two of vanilla ice-cream is a delicious addition. Berries are ideal when fresh, however frozen raspberries, black or blueberries are also great.

1 banana, peeled and roughly chopped
150g berries, frozen or fresh, defrosted
1 orange, juiced
200g yoghurt, natural or fruit
1 cup milk (cow, oat, brown rice or coconut)
1–2 scoops ice-cream (optional)

Place the chopped banana, berries, orange juice and yoghurt into a blender and pulse until smooth. Add the milk and ice-cream (if using) and pulse until combined. Pour into 2 tumblers.

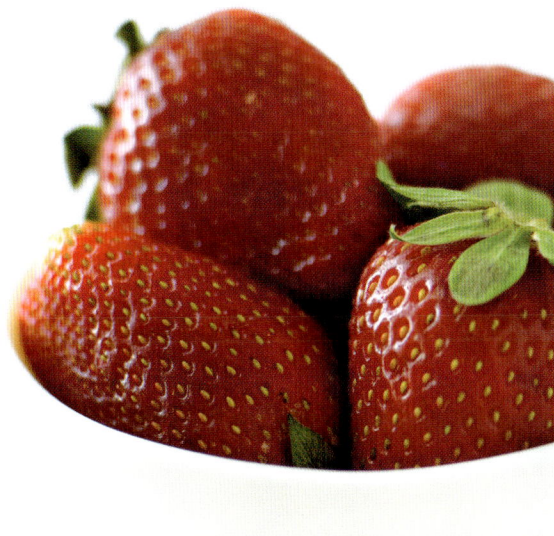

breakfast smoothie

This smoothie provides protein, calcium and fibre, all in one glass!

2 cups milk (cow, oat, brown rice or coconut)
3/4 cup plain yoghurt
1 tablespoon wheatgerm
1 tablespoon oatbran
1 egg
1 teaspoon vanilla extract
1–2 teaspoons honey (optional)
pinch of cinnamon

Place all the ingredients (except cinnamon) in a blender or food processor. Blend until smooth. Pour into 2 glasses and sprinkle with the cinnamon.

raspberry and strawberry smoothie

Frozen berries are great for those times when fresh fruit is not available or you're hankering for a taste of summer!

200g raspberries, defrosted
200g strawberries, defrosted
1 ruby grapefruit, juiced
400ml milk (cow, oat, brown rice or coconut)
1–2 scoops ice-cream (optional)

Blend the fruit, juice and coconut milk together until smooth. Add a scoopful of vanilla or strawberry ice-cream for an indulgent change and a mint leaf for decoration. Makes 2 glasses.

fruit lassi

Use either whole milk yoghurt or low-fat yoghurt to make these delicious drinks.

1 cup plain yoghurt
1 banana or other soft fruit like peach, apricot, nectarine or mango
3 cups ice-cold water
cinnamon or nutmeg to serve

Blend ingredients until smooth and serve with cinnamon or nutmeg sprinkled on top. Serves 2.

sweet lassi

1 cup plain yoghurt
3 cups ice-cold water
apple syrup to taste
1 tablespoon coconut cream
few drops rose essence
2 tablespoons orange blossom water

Blend ingredients and serve in 2 cold glasses.

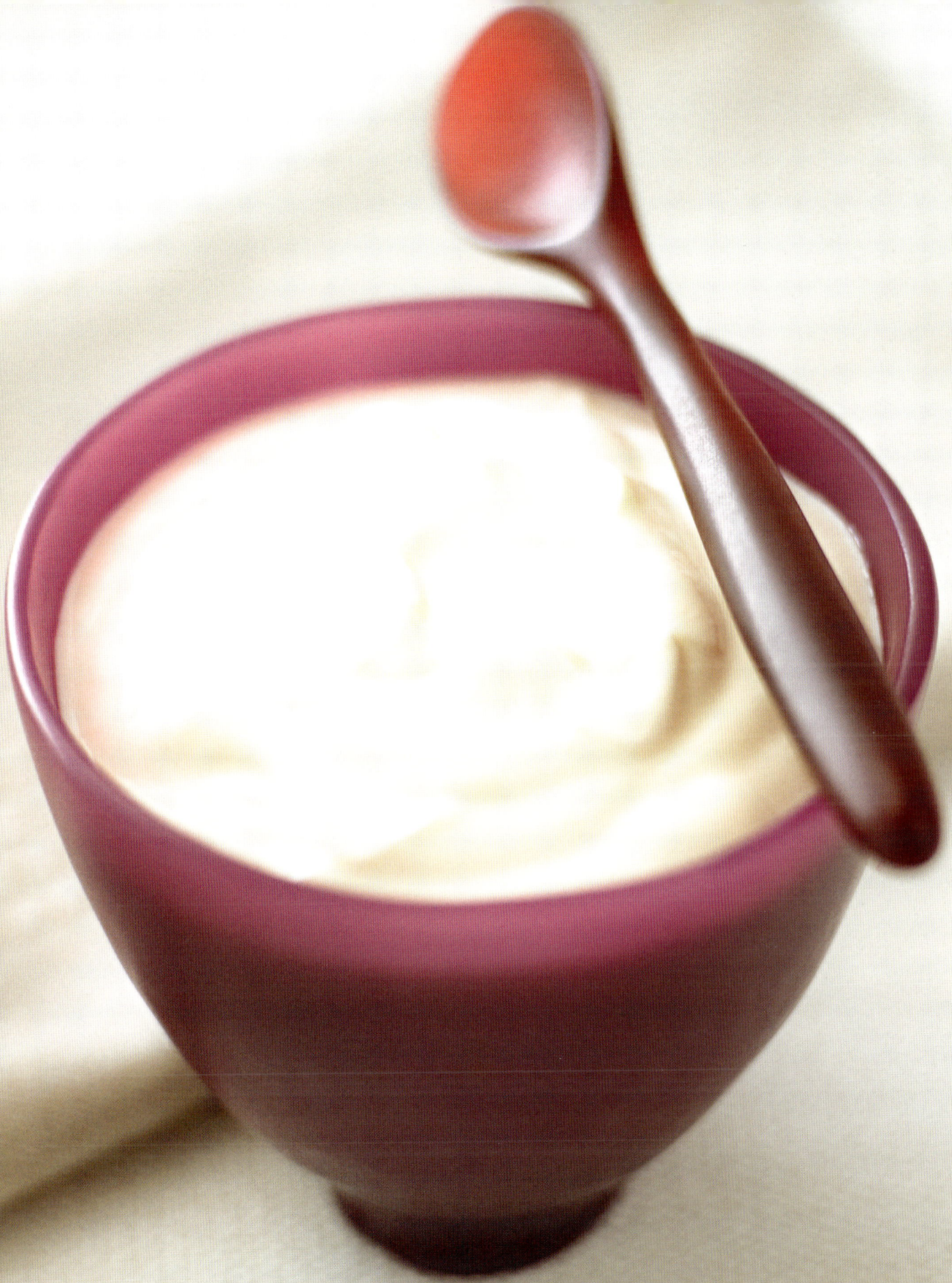

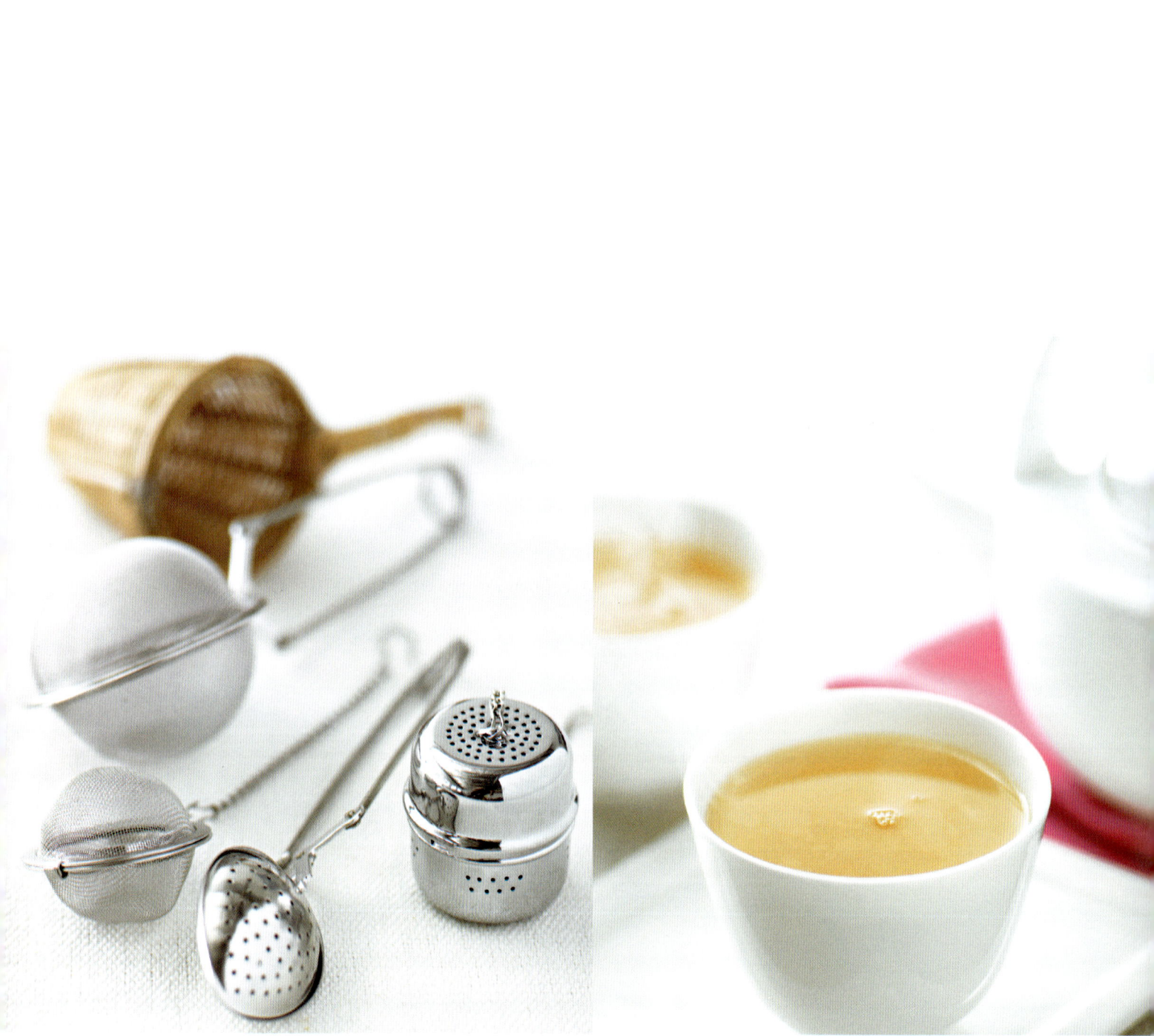

ginger tea

This tea is also delicious made with fresh lime juice instead of lemon. For a speedy variation, just pop slices of ginger and lemon or lime in a cup and pour over boiling water.

1/4 cup sliced ginger
4 cups boiling water
1 tablespoon lemon juice
1 tablespoon honey (optional)

Place the sliced ginger into a saucepan and add the boiling water. Simmer over a low heat for 10 minutes. Stir through the lemon juice and honey (if using) and pour into heatproof glasses or cups. Sip slowly. Serves 4.

Ginger tea is both refreshing and very soothing for upset stomachs.
It is also a warming drink when you feel cold from 'the bones out'.

spiced ginger tea

This is a lovely variation on the ginger tea recipe. Don't be scared off by the inclusion of garlic as its flavour doesn't dominate and it is great for warding off colds.

1 litre water
2 lemons, juiced
1 ginger tea bag
1 clove garlic, finely chopped
3cm piece ginger, finely chopped
1/2 teaspoon cinnamon
2 teaspoons honey

Place the water in a saucepan and bring to the boil. Add the lemon juice, tea bag, garlic, ginger, cinnamon and honey. Reduce the heat and simmer for 5 minutes. Strain and serve. This is also delicious as a cold drink or frozen into iceblocks. Serves 2.

peppermint and green tea

Green tea is well known for its antioxidant qualities and combined with mint leaves it makes a most refreshing tea. You may find that the Japanese varieties of green tea have a smoother flavour than the Chinese ones. Green tea contains catechin, vitamins B, C and E, plant pigments, antioxidants, fluorine and saponin.

2 teaspoons green tea leaves (or 2 tea bags)
2 tablespoons fresh peppermint leaves, or 2 tea bags
2–3 cups boiling water

Place the tea leaves and mint leaves in a warm teapot and cover with boiling water. Leave to infuse for a few minutes and pour into small tea cups or glasses. Serves 2.

chamomile and orange tea

Chamomile tea is calming and soothing, helps promote sleep and aids digestion. It is also a lovely drink to sip on throughout the day.

1 teaspoon chamomile tea (or tea bag)
1 cup boiling water
1 tablespoon orange juice

Infuse the tea in boiling water for 2 minutes. Pour into a cup or glass and stir through the orange juice. Serves 1.

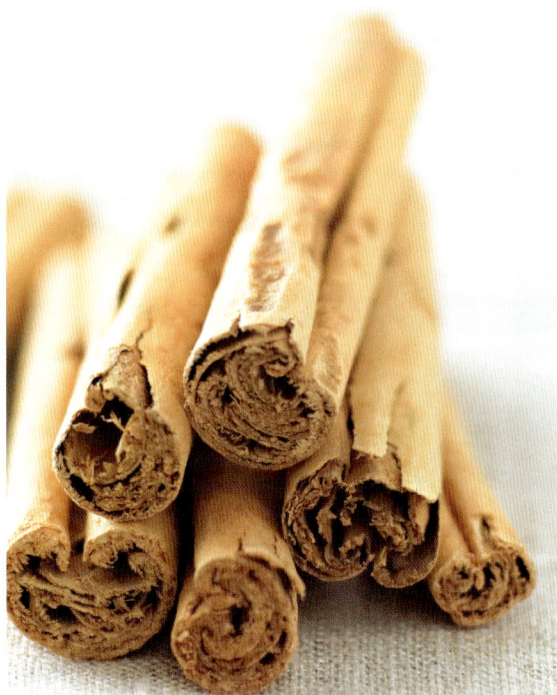

cardamom and orange tea

While this tea is fabulous to drink hot, it is also very refreshing if served chilled in a tall glass with ice. Substitute the orange juice with ruby red grapefruit juice for one of the most refreshing and thirst-quenching drinks you can make. It's also delicious made into ice cubes.

2 cardamom pods
3 oranges, juiced
2 strips orange rind
1 cinnamon stick
2 cups water

Use the flat edge of a heavy knife to crack open the cardamom pods. Place in a saucepan with the orange juice, rind and cinnamon stick. Add the water and bring to the boil then turn off the heat. Leave to infuse for about 2 hours. Strain and serve hot or chilled with ice. Serves 2.

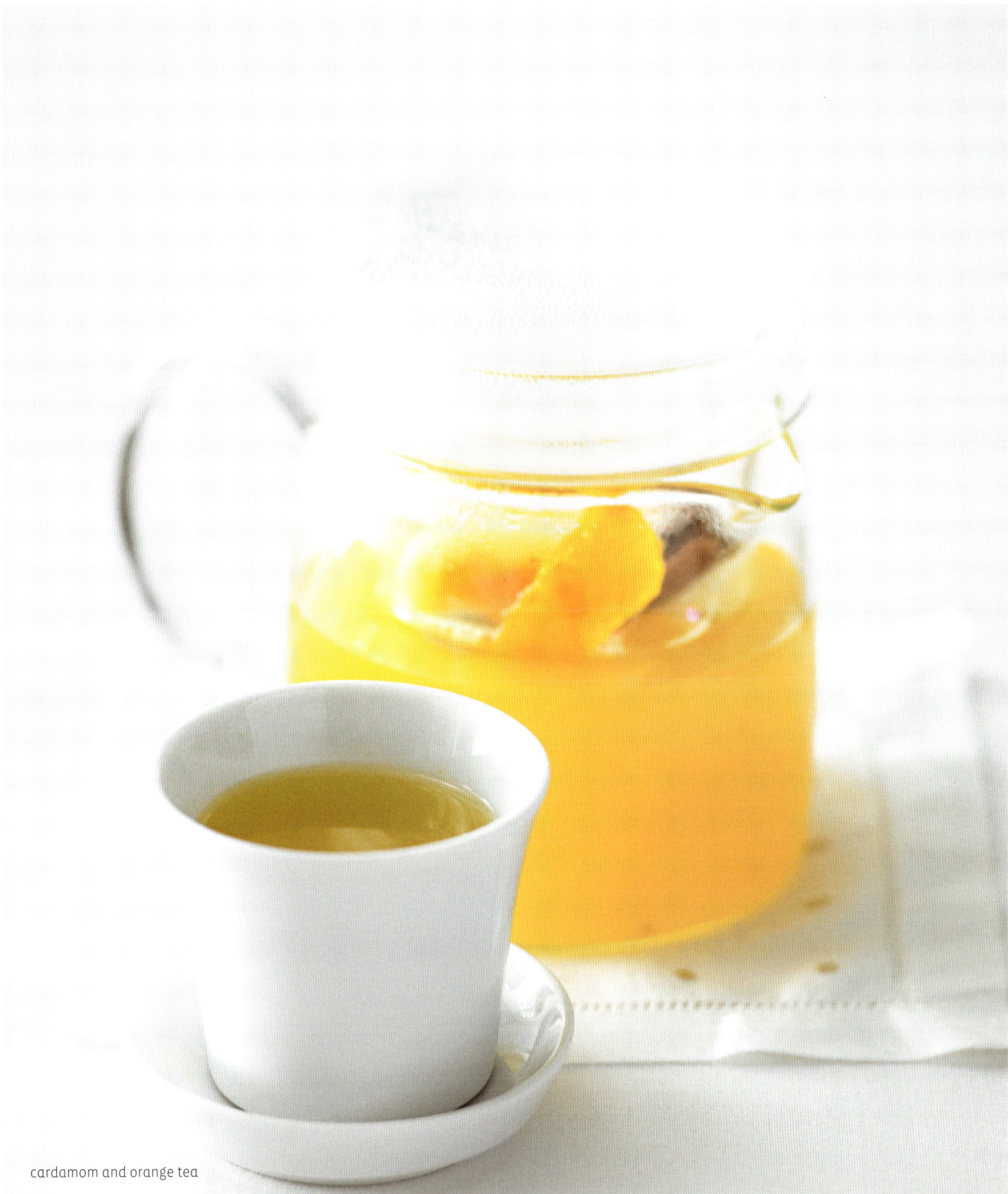

cardamom and orange tea

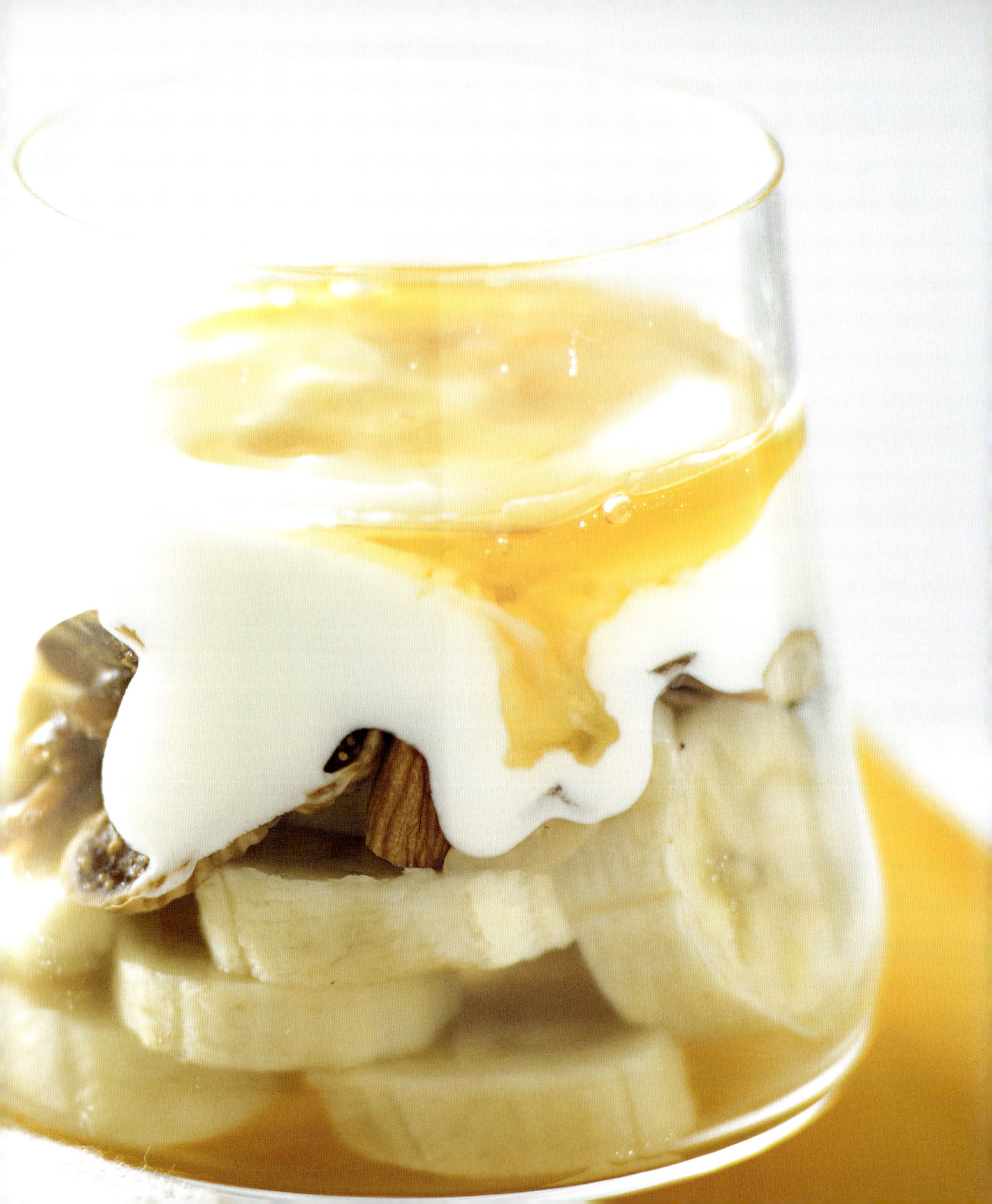

Breakfast

breakfast

The first meal of the day needs to provide sustaining nutrition to carry us into the activities of the day, and fibre to act like a 'broom' through our digestive system.

WE EACH HAVE different dietary requirements depending on our levels of activity, individual likes and dislikes, cultural background, the amount of time we choose to devote to food preparation and our emotional and psychological state. This is why I believe that no single diet is suitable for all people. It's important to listen to your own body and find foods that work for you.

A good start to the day is a cleansing drink that stimulates the body's production of enzymes and prepares our stomach for digestion. Many people like to wake up their digestive system with a glass of pure warm water with half a lemon or grapefruit squeezed into it half an hour before eating. A vegetable or fresh fruit juice is also an excellent way to start the day. You'll find plenty of suggestions for delicious juices in the previous chapter.

If you find it difficult to eat a hearty breakfast, then consider taking some nutritious, tasty bits and pieces with you in the morning. You'll then be prepared to meet any mid-morning hunger pangs with some wholesome foods rather than reaching for sweet or salty things. A couple of pieces of fresh fruit, some seeds, nuts, dried fruits and yoghurt are all simple to prepare and carry with you.

Gradually reduce any sugary, over-processed cereals and manufactured breakfast products from your pantry. And start avoiding foods that contain unnecessary chemicals, sugar and white flour and replace them with rolled oats, whole grains, seeds, nuts and dried fruits. Stock up with your preferred type of milk and plenty of seasonal fruits and you'll have all you need for an energising breakfast.

The recipes that follow will give you a great choice of tempting ideas. We tend to get into a routine where we eat the same breakfast each day. On the weekends or more leisurely mornings, you might like to try some of these ideas, or make a batch of delicious muesli so you always have it on hand.

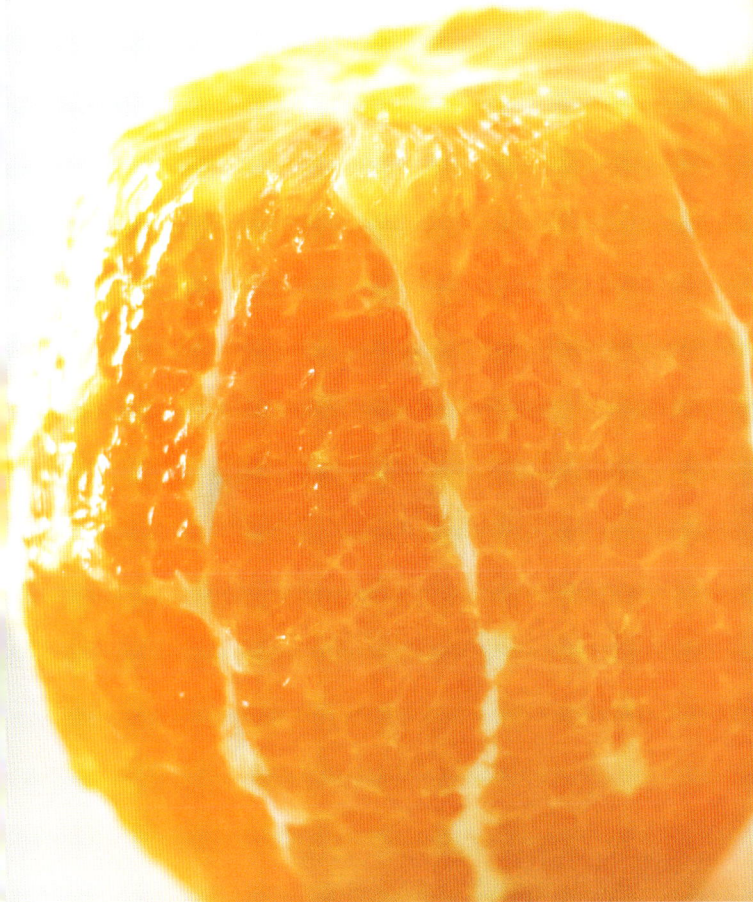
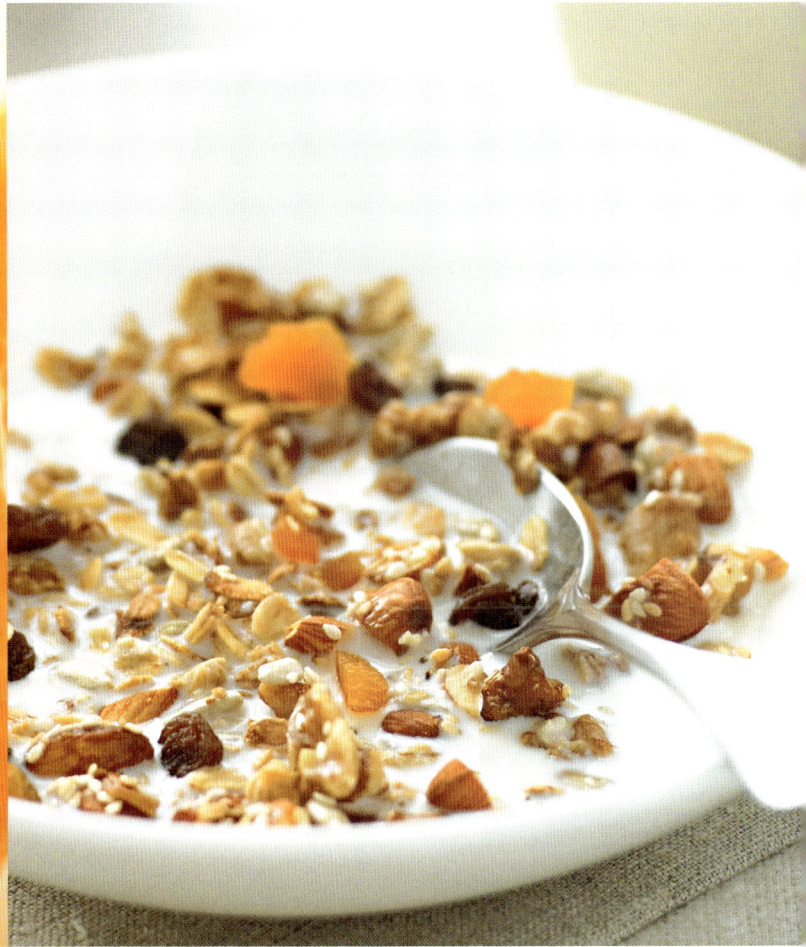

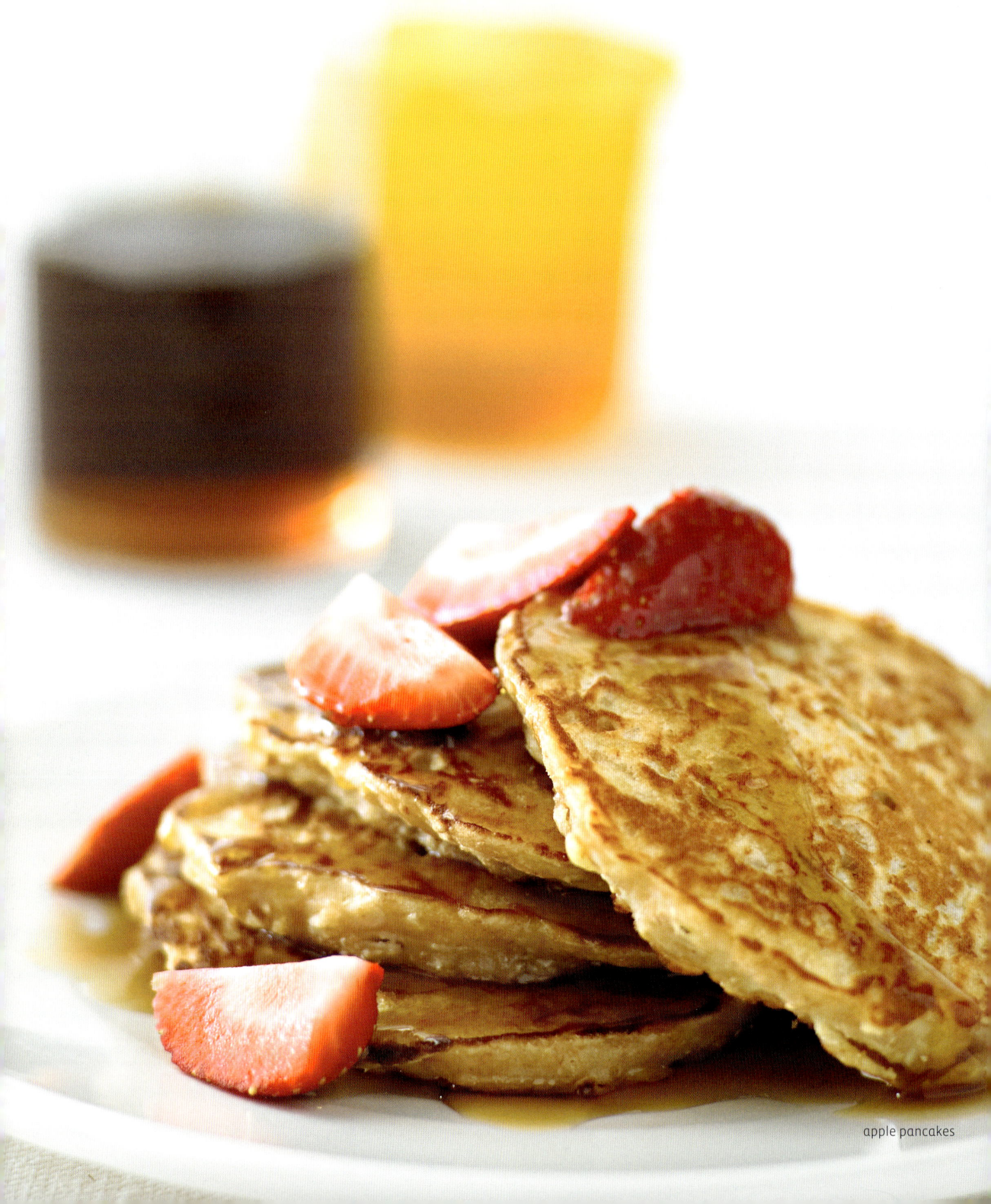

apple pancakes

date porridge

Porridge is a staple breakfast at the Quest for Life Centre. Oats are the perfect breakfast as they slowly release energy into our bodies throughout the morning. Adding chopped dried dates provides natural sweetness and is delicious.

1 1/2 cups rolled oats
1 1/2 cups pure water
1 1/2 cups milk (cow, oat, brown rice or coconut) or water
4 dates, pitted and cut into slivers
pinch of cinnamon

Place the oats in a small saucepan and add the water and milk. Cook over a medium heat for 3–4 minutes or until the oats have thickened and cooked. Stir through the dates and spoon into 2 warm bowls. Sprinkle with ground cinnamon. Add your preferred milk to taste. Serves 2.

apple pancakes

These pancakes will be popular with everyone. Other fruits such as blueberries, pears or chopped banana can be used instead of apple. Always use ripe and seasonal fruit to maximise the flavour — fruit in season is the most economical as well.

1 cup wholemeal flour
1/2 teaspoon baking powder
1 egg
1 cup milk (cow, brown rice, oat or coconut)
1 tablespoon warm honey
2 apples, cored and grated
coconut or extra-virgin olive oil or ghee
maple syrup to serve

Place the flour and baking powder in a mixing bowl. Lightly beat together the egg, milk and warm honey in a jug and gradually pour into the flour, while whisking, to form a smooth batter. Fold through the grated apple.

Heat a frying pan and add a small amount of oil or ghee, just to coat. Pour in 1/4 cupfuls of batter and cook over medium heat, turning once, until the pancakes are golden on both sides. Remove pancakes from the pan and keep warm while cooking the remaining mixture. Serve drizzled with maple syrup. Serves 4.

rainbow muesli

Rainbows have a special significance at the Quest for Life Centre and we also like to use their many colours in our food. Make yourself a rainbow at the beginning of the day with this delicious muesli.

$2/3$ cup rolled oats
1 cup milk (cow, brown rice, oat, coconut) or apple juice or water
1 apple, cored and grated
$1/3$ cup natural yoghurt (sheep's yoghurt is delicious while goat's milk has a stronger flavour)
chopped seasonal fruits in all the colours of the rainbow (strawberries, cherries, papaya, oranges, apricots, bananas, kiwifruit, grapes and blueberries etc.)

Combine the oats and grated apple and your choice of fruit and top with your favourite milk and yoghurt. Serves 2.

lemon pikelets with raspberry sauce

This winning combination of flavours with real zing can be cooked ahead of time and warmed when needed.

2 cups raspberries, fresh or frozen, defrosted
2 tablespoons lemon juice
1 tablespoon honey or golden syrup
1 cup self-raising flour
3 teaspoons grated lemon zest
2 tablespoons raw or palm sugar
1 egg, lightly beaten
$2/3$ cup milk (cow, coconut, brown rice or oat)
coconut or extra-virgin olive oil or ghee

Place half the raspberries in a food processor or blender and add the lemon juice and honey or golden syrup. Blend until smooth. Combine the puree with the remaining raspberries and set aside while you make the pikelets.

Combine the flour, lemon zest and raw or palm sugar in a mixing bowl. Whisk together the egg and milk and stir into the flour mixture until smooth.

Heat a large frying pan. Brush with oil or ghee and spoon tablespoons of the pikelet mixture into the pan. Cook for 2 minutes or until bubbles appear on the top side of the pikelet. Turn over and cook for another 30 seconds. Keep warm while you cook the remaining mixture or let cool and store for later use.

Serve a stack of pikelets for each person and spoon over the raspberry sauce. Serves 3–4.

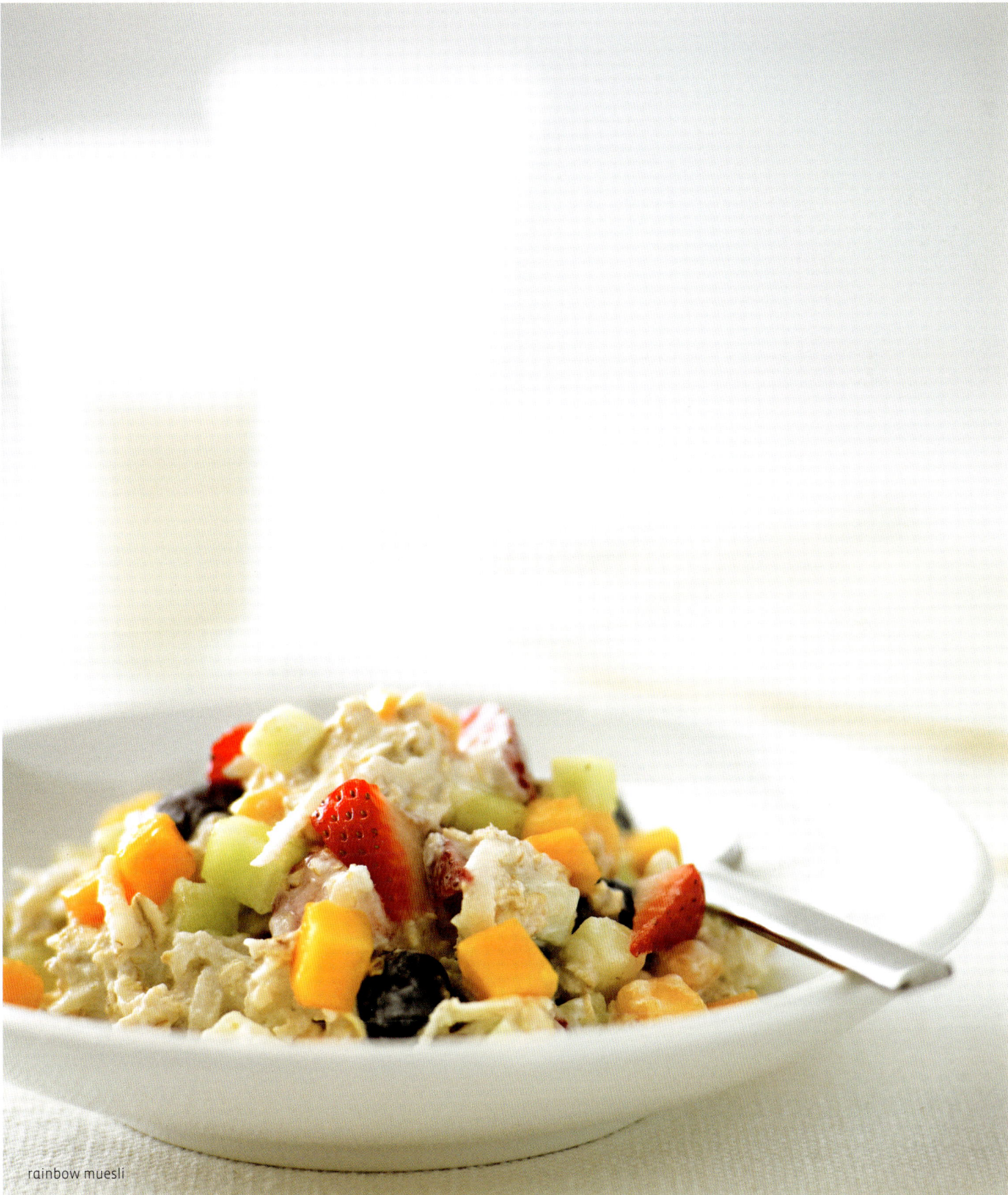

rainbow muesli

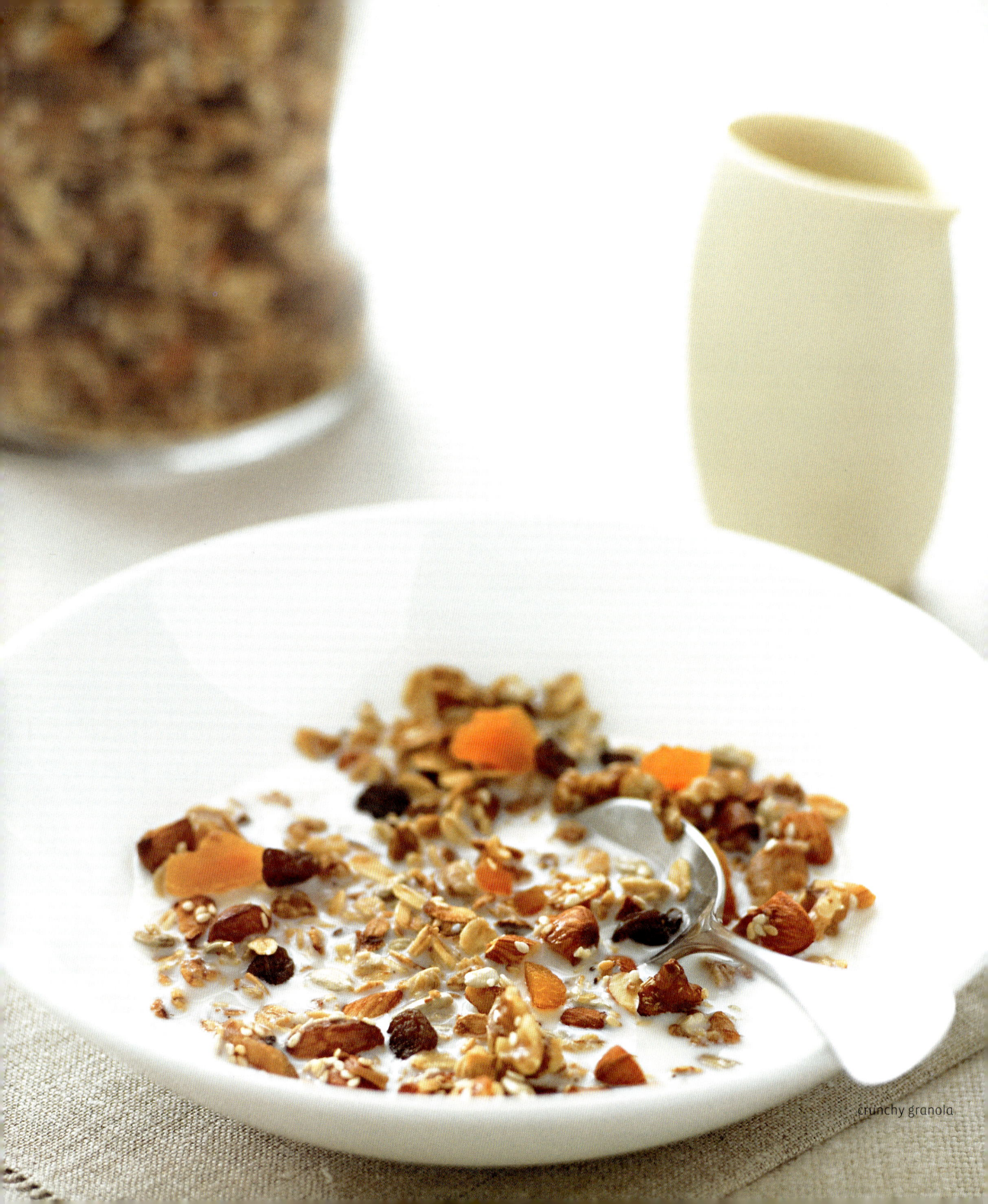

crunchy granola

crunchy granola

Making your own granola is so rewarding and it tastes much better than bought varieties. It is very easy to make and the only effort is getting to the shop to buy the ingredients.

2 cups rolled oats
1/4 cup sunflower seeds
2 tablespoons sesame seeds
1/2 cup raw almonds, chopped
1/2 cup raw walnuts, roughly chopped
1/4 cup maple syrup
1/4 cup honey
1/3 cup chopped dried apricots
1/3 cup sultanas

Preheat the oven to 180°C and line 2 baking trays with non-stick baking paper. Combine the oats, sunflower seeds, sesame seeds, almonds and walnuts in a large mixing bowl.

Gently heat the maple syrup and honey together and pour over the oat mixture. Toss together using a couple of metal spoons and then spread the mixture evenly over the 2 baking trays. Bake in the oven for 20–30 minutes or until evenly golden. You will need to rearrange the granola on the baking trays every 5 minutes so that it cooks evenly.

Allow the granola to cool then fold through the apricots and sultanas. Store in an airtight container. Serve with your favourite milk. Makes 500g.

NON-STICK PANS

Have you noticed that after using a non-stick pan for a while the surface begins to come away even if you've been careful to use the right implements? The substance used to make pans non-stick is a carcinogenic chemical that is designed for convenience but not for ingestion into the human body. Choose good quality stainless steel, enamel, ceramic or glass cookware to bake and cook in instead.

breakfast muffins

These are perfect if you are feeling particularly organised in the morning. Otherwise you can get all the dry ingredients in the bowl the night before if you want to make life easy. The seeds in these muffins are a fabulous source of concentrated protein and fibre.

2 cups wholemeal flour
2 teaspoons baking powder
1/3 cup raw sugar (optional)
1/4 cup sultanas
2 tablespoons sunflower seeds
1 tablespoon sesame seeds
1 cup milk (cow, brown rice, oat or coconut)
50g unsalted butter, ghee, coconut or extra-virgin olive oil
1 egg
1 tablespoon pumpkin seeds

Preheat the oven to 200°C. Lightly brush a 12 hole 1/2 cup muffin tin with melted butter, ghee or oil. Sift the flour and baking powder into a large bowl. Add the raw sugar (if using), sultanas and sunflower and sesame seeds.

Combine the milk, egg and melted butter, oil or ghee and pour into the flour mixture. Stir until just combined. Spoon the mixture into the muffin tin and scatter with the pumpkin seeds. Bake for 20 minutes or until cooked.

Remove from the oven and let stand for 5 minutes to firm up. Cool slightly on a wire rack before devouring. If you want to freeze or store them let them cool completely. Makes 12.

This soft pink compote is a lovely way to greet the day. Rhubarb is easy to grow in the garden and provides a never-ending supply for the kitchen.

pear and rhubarb compote

If you think you don't like rhubarb, you might be pleasantly surprised by this combination. Try making the night before and place in a ceramic dish in the fridge.

4 pears, cored, peeled and cut into wedges
1 bunch rhubarb, trimmed, washed
   and cut into 4cm lengths
2 tablespoons honey

Place the pear wedges and rhubarb in a saucepan and add a couple of tablespoons of water. Gently cook, covered, over medium heat for 6–8 minutes or until the rhubarb is tender. Be careful not to overcook. Stir through the honey. Serve warm or at room temperature. Serves 4.

banana, nut and fig yoghurt

This is a lovely way to treat yourself to a healthy variety of food types for breakfast.

4 bananas
$1/3$ cup assorted raw nuts (almonds, walnuts, pecans,
   macadamias etc.)
4 soft, dried figs, thinly sliced
400g plain yoghurt
2 tablespoons clear honey

Peel and slice the bananas into 4 tumblers. Roughly chop the nuts and combine with the sliced figs. Sprinkle on top of the banana. Top with yoghurt and a dessertspoon of honey. Serves 4.

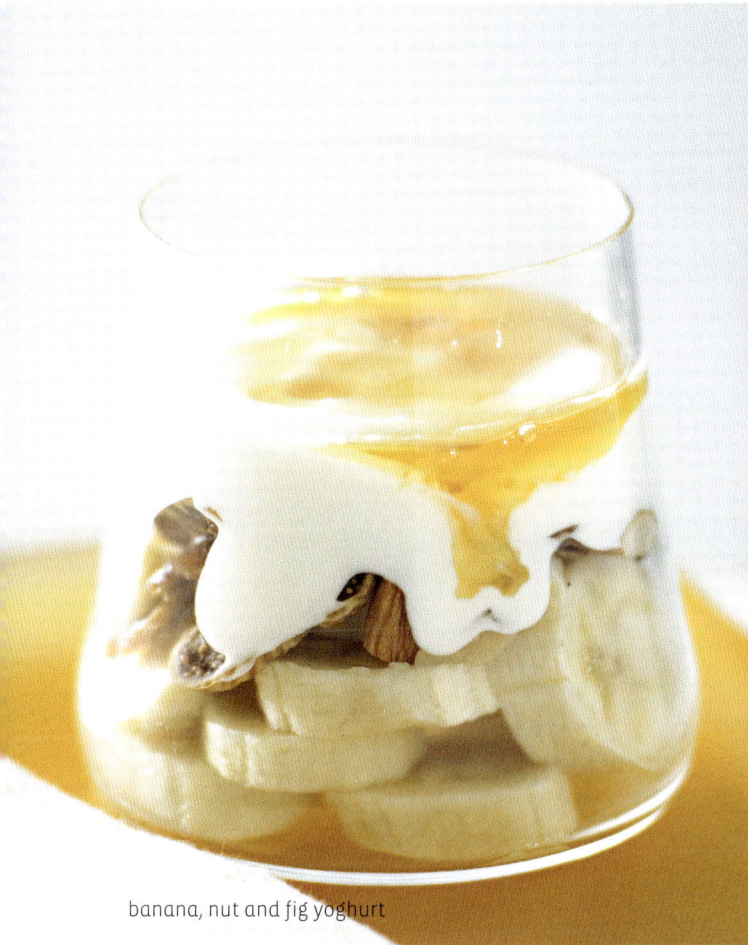

banana, nut and fig yoghurt

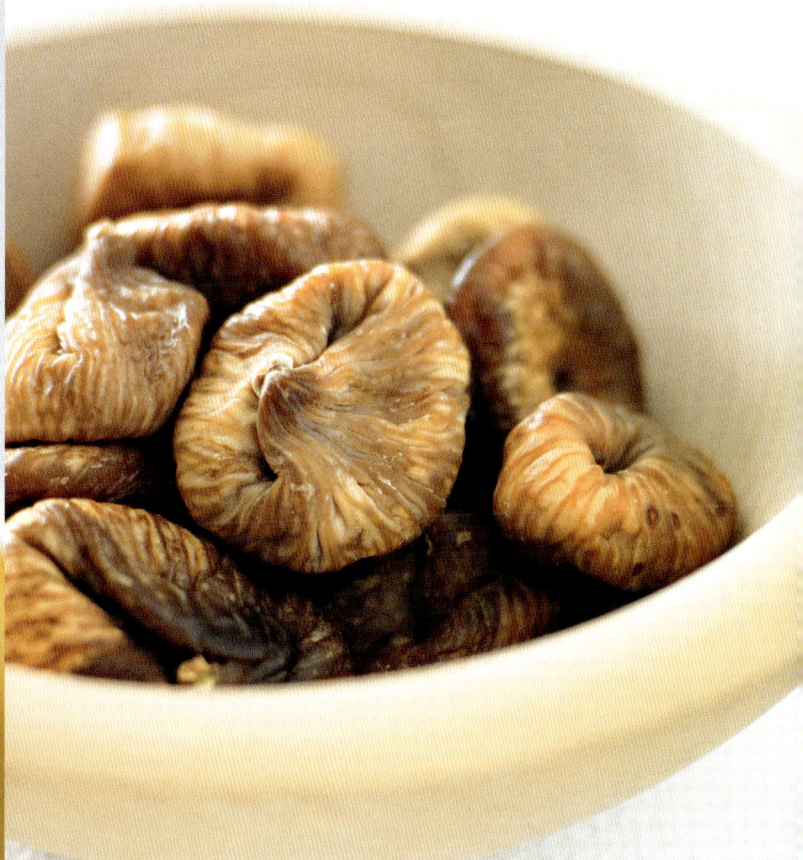

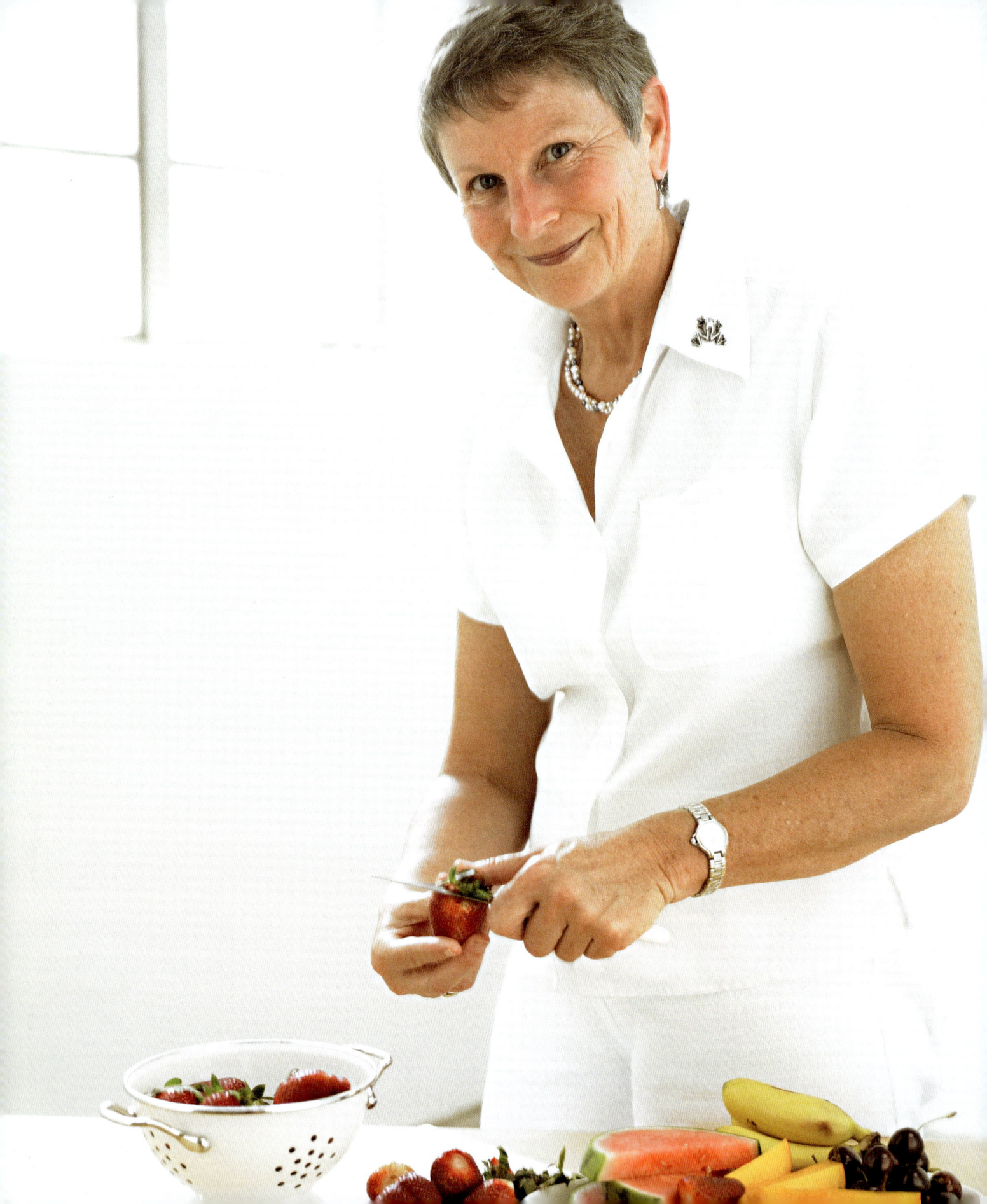

rainbow fruit platter

This is more a serving suggestion than an actual recipe and follows the rainbow theme again. Use fresh seasonal fruits for their flavour.

seasonal fruits of all different colours,
    peeled and sliced if necessary
1/3 cup shredded dried coconut
plain yoghurt to serve

Preheat the oven to 180°C. Arrange the coconut on a baking tray and cook for 5 minutes or until golden. Set a timer as it's easy to forget!

Arrange the fruit on 4 serving plates or on a platter. Sprinkle over the toasted coconut and serve with yoghurt. Serves 4.

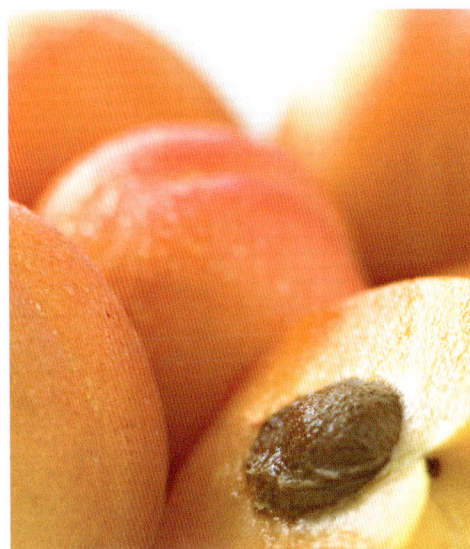

apricot and date bread

To make this delicious bread, you need to buy the bran cereal which looks like worms(!), not the flakes. Serve fresh or toasted. It is so flavoursome, it doesn't really need butter or jam.

1 cup spelt all-bran or Kelloggs All-Bran Original cereal
90g pitted dates, chopped
175g dried apricots, chopped
1 cup pureed apple (or apple sauce)
1 cup milk (cow, oat, brown rice or coconut)
1 1/2 cups wholemeal self-raising flour

Place the All-Bran, dates and apricots and pureed apple in a large bowl. Stir through the milk and soak for 2 hours.

Preheat the oven to 160°C. Line a 20x10cm loaf tin with non-stick baking paper. Fold the flour into the All-Bran mixture and combine well. Spoon the mixture into the prepared loaf tin. Bake for 1 hour or until cooked (when a skewer inserted into the centre comes out clean). Place on a wire rack to cool.

avocado and pear on toast

This combination may sound strange, but it is delicious and takes just a couple of minutes to make.

4 slices wholegrain or sourdough toast
1 ripe avocado, mashed
1 pear, cored and sliced
black pepper

Toast the bread until golden. Pile the mashed avocado on the toast and top with slices of pear. Grind over some black pepper and tuck in. Serves 2.

cherry tomatoes on toast

Cherry tomatoes just burst with flavour, colour and goodness. You can top this with a poached egg or two to add some protein.

1 tablespoon extra-virgin olive oil or coconut oil
500g red and yellow cherry tomatoes, halved
3 teaspoons apple cider vinegar
2 tablespoons chopped fresh herbs
   (basil, chives, parsley etc.)
sourdough or wholegrain toast

Heat a frying pan and warm the oil. Add the tomatoes and cook for 2–3 minutes or until soft. Stir through the vinegar and chopped herbs and serve on toast. Serves 4.

HAPPY EGGS

Happy, healthy hens lay happy, healthy eggs! How can a highly stressed chicken kept in an artificially lit building produce a wholesome egg? It can't! Hens raised in humane conditions and natural surroundings where they have sunshine, fresh air and a varied, and preferably organic, diet produce eggs that have increased flavour and colour. Likewise, if you choose to eat red or white meats, ensure that the animals were raised humanely and in a healthy open-range environment.

french toast

This is a huge favourite with young and old and is a hearty start to the day. You can use Turkish bread, wholegrain bread or sourdough.

8 slices of bread
4 eggs, lightly beaten
1/2 cup milk (cow, oat, brown rice or coconut)
1 teaspoon vanilla extract
4 teaspoons sesame or extra-virgin olive or coconut oil
1/3 cup maple syrup

Whisk together the eggs, milk and vanilla. Heat a large frying pan and add a teaspoon of the oil. Dip 2 slices of bread into the egg mixture and fully coat both sides. Add to the frying pan and cook on each side until golden and the egg is set. Repeat with the remaining slices of bread.

Serve cut into triangles and drizzle with maple syrup. Serves 4.

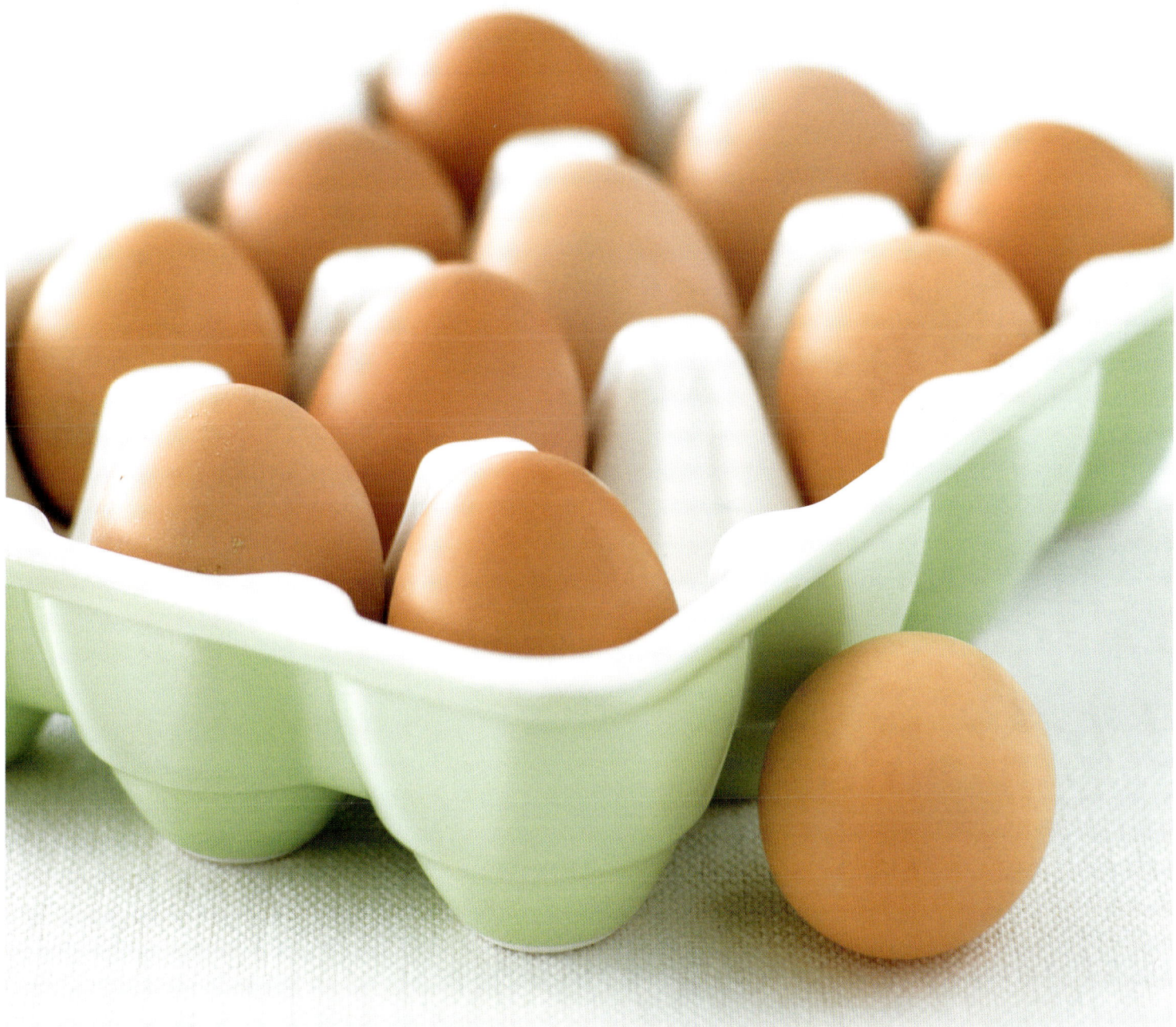

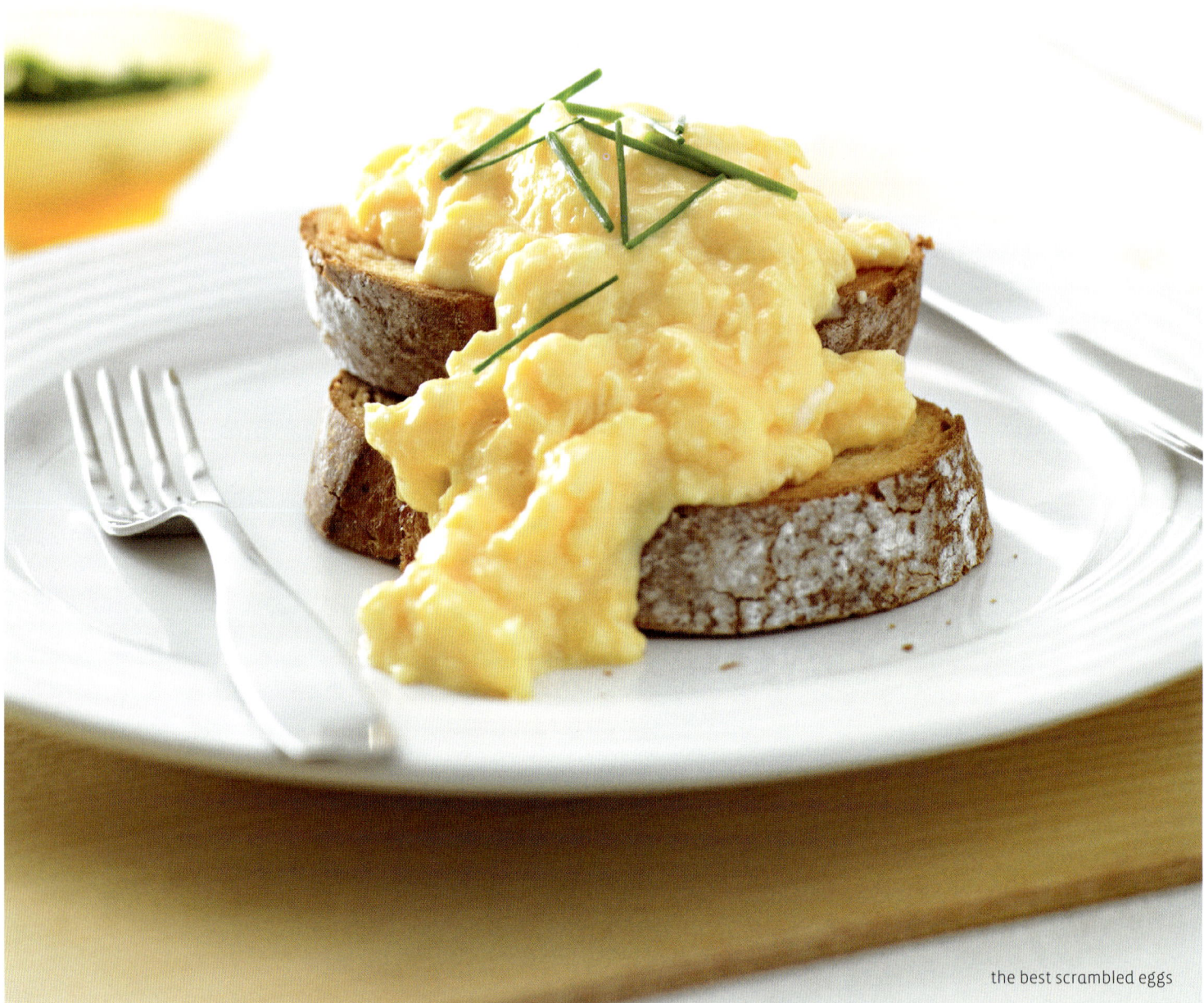

herb omelettes with mushrooms

Omelettes are so easy to make yet feel somewhat special. You can make this omelette with just the herbs or substitute the cooked mushrooms with some diced tomato, steamed asparagus or corn.

2 cups sliced mushrooms
2 teaspoons unsalted butter, ghee,
  extra-virgin olive oil or coconut oil
6 eggs
1 tablespoon fresh chopped herbs (chives, parsley etc.)

Heat a small frying pan until very hot. Add the mushrooms and a few teaspoons of water and cook while stirring until they are browned and soft. Remove from heat and add the herbs to the mushrooms to allow them to soften. Remove from the pan and keep warm while you cook the omelettes.

Beat 3 eggs and 2 teaspoons of herbs in a small bowl. Place the pan back on the heat. Add half the butter, ghee or oil, swirl around and pour the egg mixture into the pan.

As soon as the egg mixture starts to cook, using a wooden spoon or egg slice, drag the cooked egg to the centre, allowing the uncooked egg to flow to the edges. Cook for about 2 minutes then fold the omelette in half and slide onto a warm plate. Repeat for remaining eggs. Serve with the mushrooms and herbs. Serves 2.

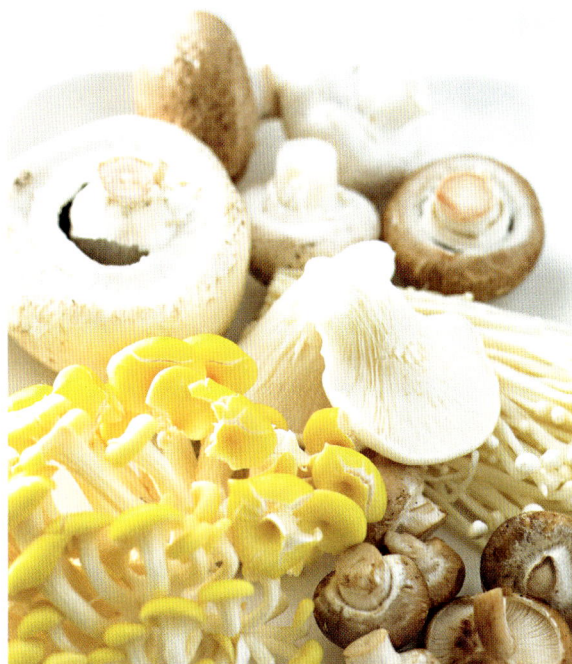

the best scrambled eggs

Scrambled eggs are fabulous emergency food for a delicious meal when you're feeling tired or when there's not much in the fridge. Try the coconut milk version for a nourishing taste sensation.

2 teaspoons unsalted butter, ghee,
  extra-virgin olive oil or coconut oil
4 eggs
$\frac{1}{4}$ cup milk (cow, oat, brown rice or coconut)
2 teaspoons chopped chives

Melt the butter, ghee or oil in a small frying or saucepan. Whisk the eggs and milk and pour into the pan. Cook for 20 seconds and then gently stir the mixture until the eggs are just set. Cooking with coconut milk will take longer for the mixture to set. You can also chop up two or three shallots and soften in the pan before adding the egg mixture. Spoon onto a warm plate and sprinkle with the chives. Serve with hot sourdough toast. Serves 2.

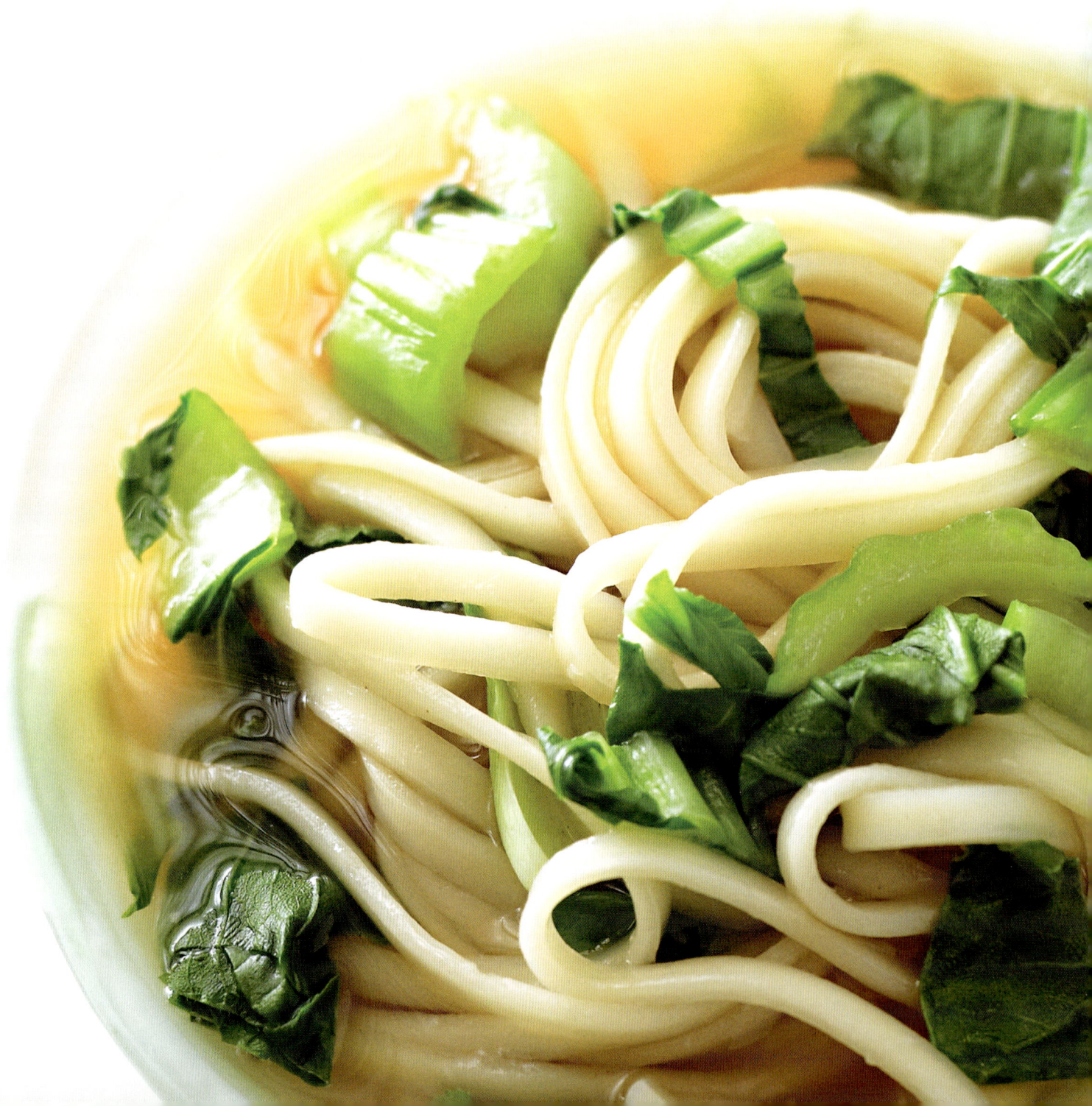

Light
Meals

light meals

At the Quest for Life Centre we have our main meal at lunchtime and keep lighter meals for the evening, as it is easier to digest a larger meal in the middle of the day when energy levels are high.

OBVIOUSLY THIS IS not possible for many people, but it is worth considering ways to eat more in the middle of the day and less at night.

Some of our favourite light meals are soups and salads. These can be made more substantial by adding bread or other carbohydrates such as basmati rice, wholemeal or seed bread, pasta or potatoes. Eat carbohydrate foods that are not overly processed, are free of additives, preservatives and colours and as wholesome and natural as possible.

Doug's soups are legendary at the Centre. Packed full of goodness and easy to eat and digest, they are a perfect light meal. Salads are also a great option and we serve these in abundance. Whatever we're eating, we aim to have a large variety of type and colour — a rainbow — of vegetables or salad ingredients on our plate at every meal.

When you buy your vegetable and salad foods, remember the importance of fresh and seasonal produce. If possible, buy organic vegetables as they are higher in fibre and flavour and have increased vitamins, minerals, antioxidants and trace elements. When it comes to salad dressings, get in the habit of making your own with cold-pressed oils, lemon juice, fresh garlic and herbs. You might like to start experimenting by adding less obvious vegetables to your salads like grated carrot, beetroot or lightly steamed snow peas, green beans, broccoli and cauliflower. Scattering some seeds over salads or a few raw chopped nuts also adds delicious flavours and nutrition.

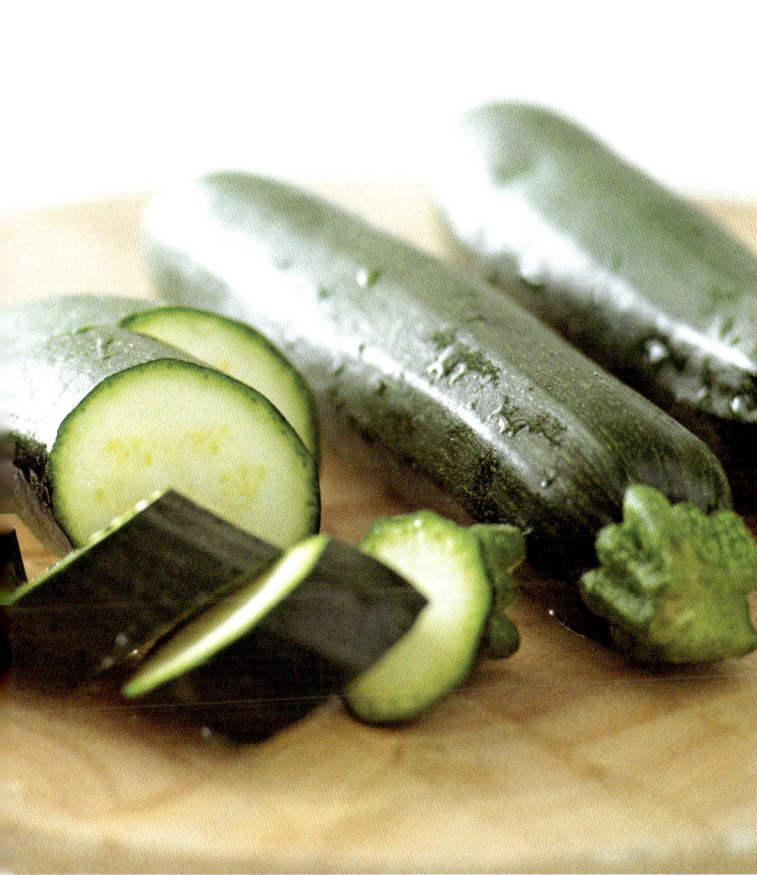
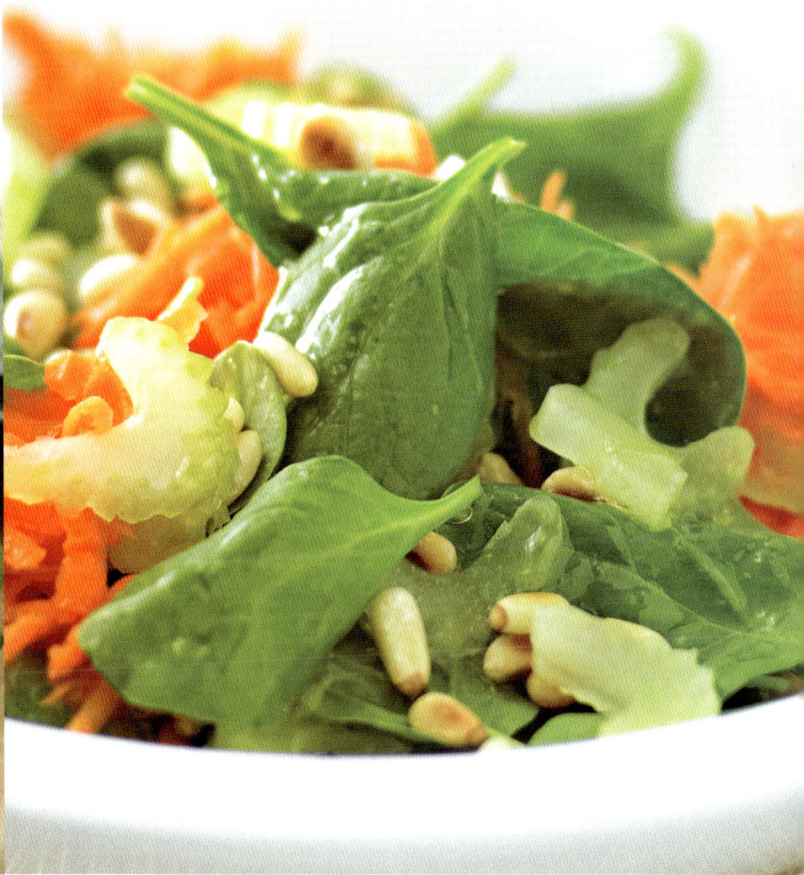

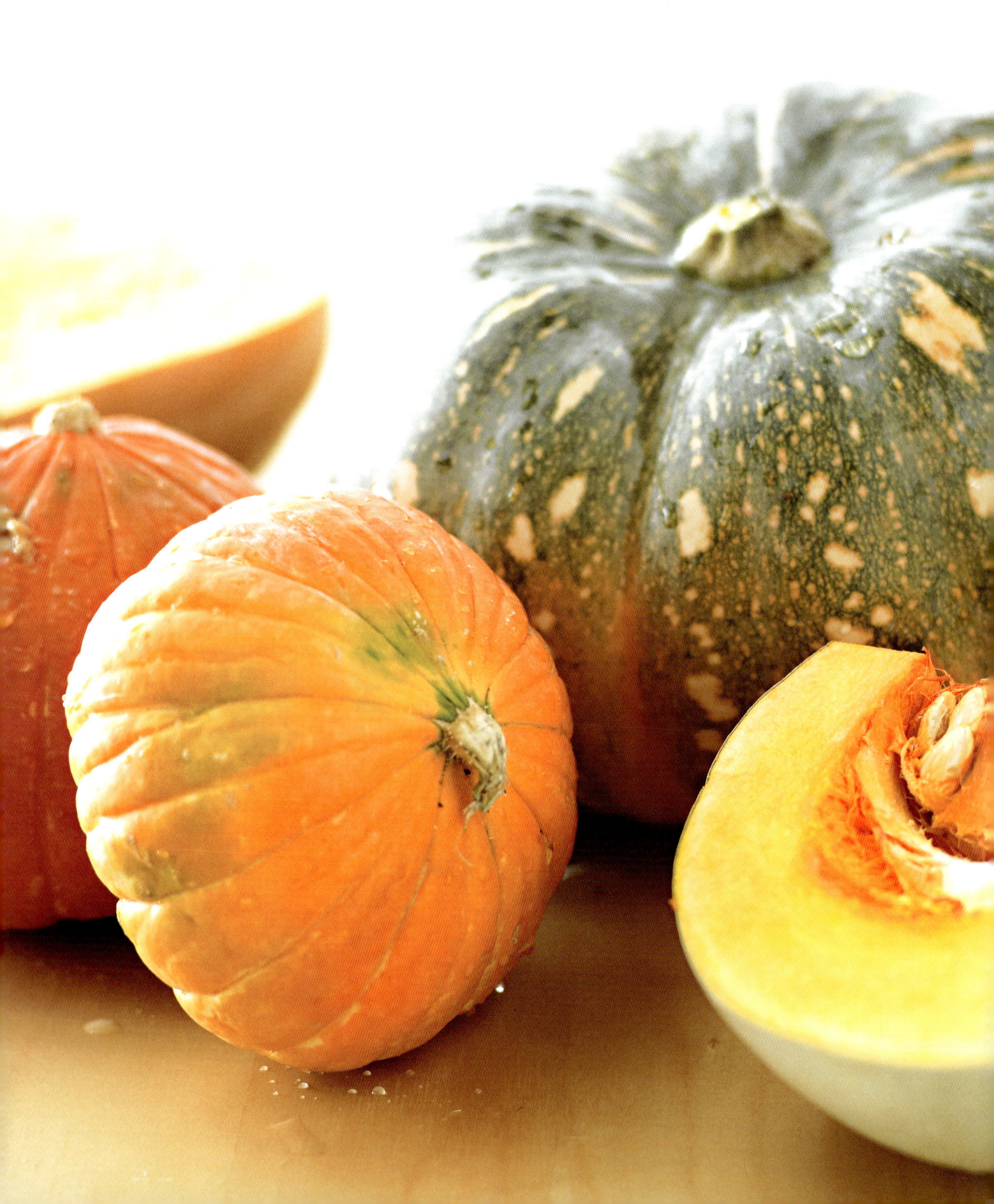

pumpkin and leek soup

It is hard to beat pumpkin soup with hot crusty sourdough bread on a chilly evening. The addition of leeks makes the soup extra smooth. If you don't want to use leeks, substitute with a large brown onion.

1 tablespoon extra-virgin olive or coconut oil
1 large leek, trimmed, cleaned and sliced
2 cloves garlic, crushed (optional)
800g peeled pumpkin, cut into chunks
6 cups vegetable stock
pinch of nutmeg
$^1/_2$ cup milk (cow, brown rice, oat or coconut)
sea salt and black pepper

Heat the oil in a large saucepan. Add the sliced leek and gently cook over low heat until soft. Cover with a lid if the leek begins to burn. Stir through the garlic (if using) and cook for another 30 seconds.

Add the pumpkin and stock and bring to the boil. Simmer for 30 minutes, partially covered, or until the pumpkin is tender. Add the nutmeg and milk and blend using either a stick blender or a food processor. Season with sea salt and freshly ground pepper and serve with warm, crusty sourdough bread. Serves 4–6.

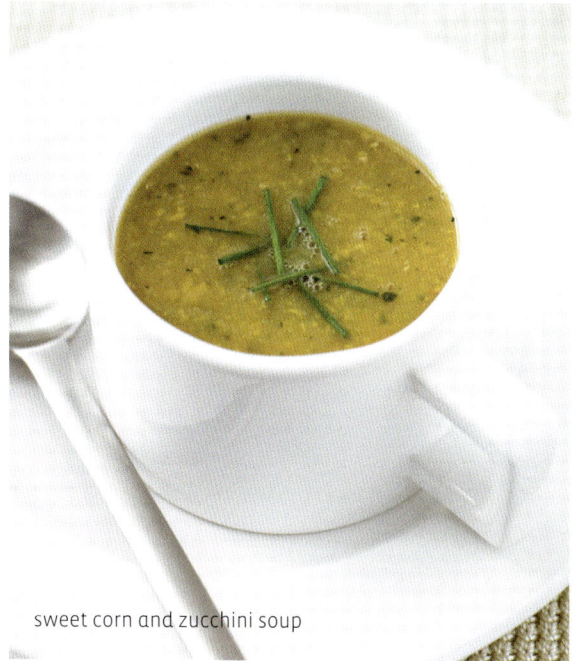

sweet corn and zucchini soup

sweet corn and zucchini soup

1 tablespoon extra-virgin olive or coconut oil
1 onion, chopped
4 corn cobs
2 zucchinis, trimmed and roughly chopped
8 cups vegetable stock
$^1/_2$ cup fresh basil leaves
sea salt and black pepper
chives for garnish

Heat the oil in a large saucepan and add the onion. Gently cook until soft and golden. Cut the corn kernels from the cobs and add to the onion along with the chopped zucchini. Cook for a couple of minutes while stirring.

Add the vegetable stock and bring to the boil. Simmer for 12 minutes or until the corn is tender and the zucchini cooked. Remove from the heat and add the basil. Blend using a stick blender or food processor. Season with sea salt and freshly ground pepper and garnish with chives. Serves 4.

vegetable and coconut soup

Lightly toasted sesame seeds can be used as a garnish instead of the coconut if you prefer.

2 tablespoons dried shredded coconut

3 teaspoons sesame oil

1 Spanish (red) onion, halved and thinly sliced

3cm piece ginger, peeled and finely chopped

$1/2$ teaspoon dried red chilli flakes (or 1 hot red chilli, seeded and chopped)

500g pumpkin, peeled, seeded and cut into 1cm cubes

3 cups vegetable stock

400ml can coconut milk

200g green beans, cut into 2cm pieces

200g snow peas, halved on the diagonal

Heat a small frying pan and lightly cook the shredded coconut until just golden. Reserve.

Heat the sesame oil in a saucepan and add the onion. Cook until soft then add the ginger and chilli. Cook for another minute. Add the pumpkin, vegetable stock and coconut milk and bring to the boil.

Reduce the heat, cover and cook for 20 minutes or until the pumpkin is tender, adding the green beans and snow peas during the last few minutes of cooking. Serve in warm bowls and sprinkle with the toasted shredded coconut. Serves 4.

udon noodle and miso soup

This tasty soup is quick to make and is very filling. You can buy udon noodles, dashi and mirin at Asian stores or some supermarkets.

6 cups water

1 tablespoon dashi granules

2 tablespoons mirin

2 tablespoons tamari or soy sauce

500g udon noodles

$1^{1}/2$ cups shredded Chinese vegetables (gai lum, baby bok choy etc.)

Place the water in a large saucepan and add the dashi, mirin and tamari. Bring slowly to the boil stirring until the dashi granules have dissolved.

Add the noodles and cook for 2 minutes. Stir through the shredded vegetables and cook until tender. Serve in large warm bowls. Adding two poached eggs creates a hearty and nutritious winter meal. Serves 4.

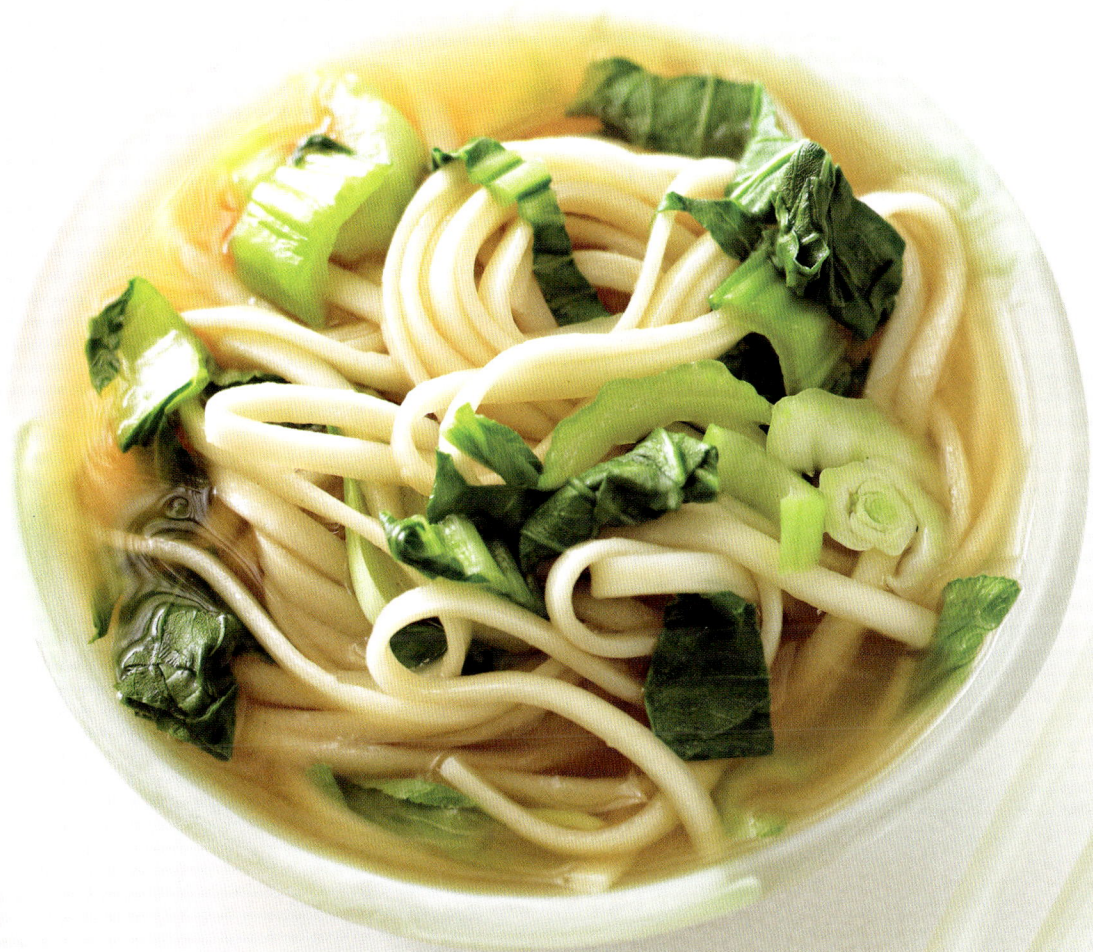

udon noodle and miso soup

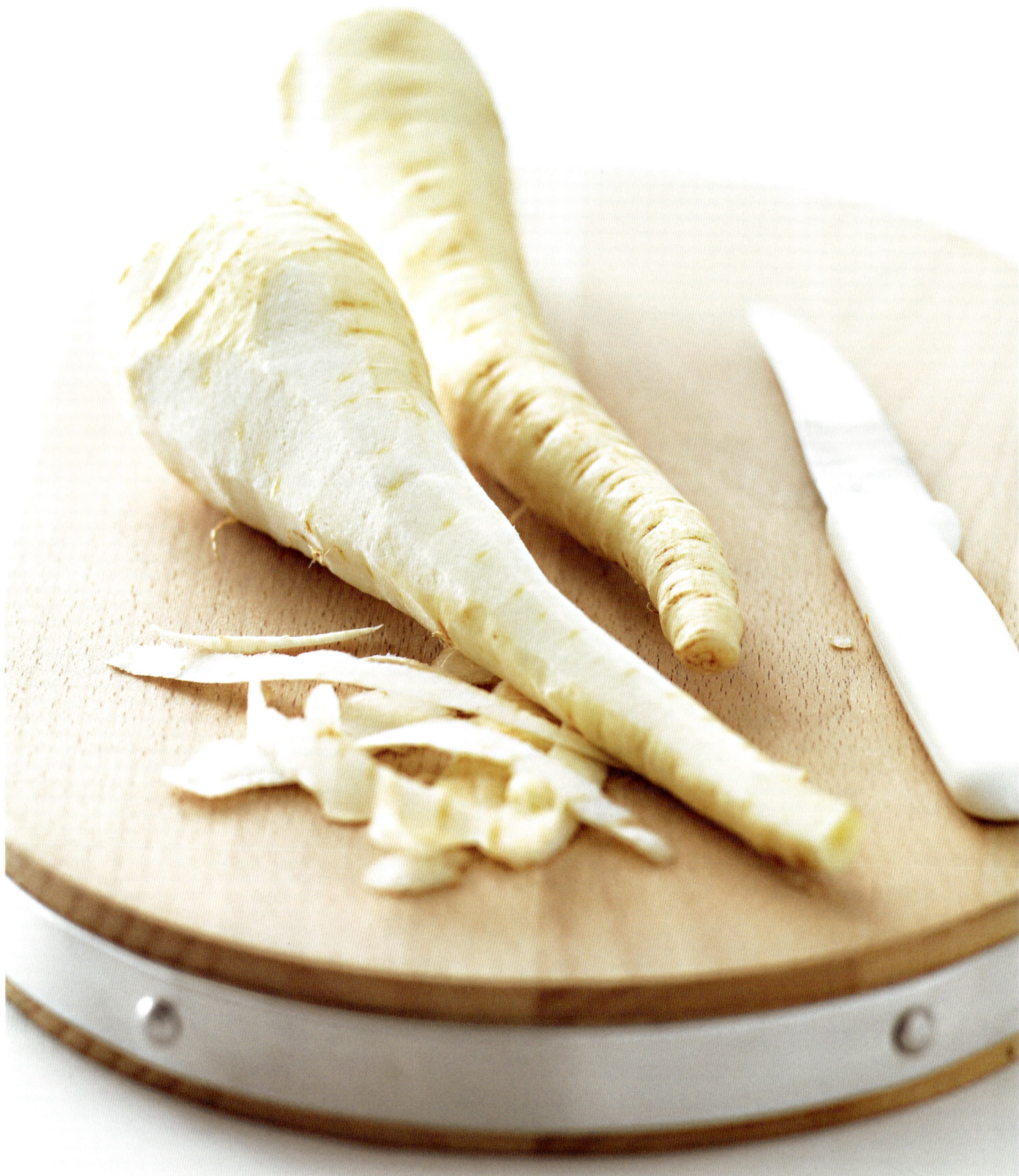

chicken soup

The trick to this soup is to make a delicious, 100 per cent natural chicken stock. This requires a bit of planning ahead but is well worth the effort. The stock can be kept in the fridge for up to 3 days or can be frozen.

stock
1 chicken
1 onion, peeled and chopped
1 carrot, sliced
1 stick celery, sliced
1 leek, cleaned and sliced
1 bay leaf
parsley stalks
6 black peppercorns

soup
2 teaspoons sesame, extra-virgin olive or coconut oil
reserved meat from chicken
1 tablespoon tamari or soy sauce
2 tablespoons chopped fresh herbs
   (parsley, chives, dill etc.)

To make the stock, cut the meat from the chicken and reserve. Place the carcass and wings in a large saucepan. Cover with 2 litres of cold spring water and bring to the boil. Lower heat until the water is just simmering and skim off fat. Add the onion, carrot, celery, leek, bay leaf, parsley stalks and black peppercorns. Gently simmer for $3\frac{1}{2}$–4 hours. Strain and put into a clean saucepan and heat to simmering point. Cool and refrigerate (or freeze if not using straight away).

To make the soup, remove skin from the reserved chicken meat and cut into bite-size pieces. Heat the oil in a frying pan and brown the chicken. Add the browned chicken to the saucepan of hot stock and simmer for 10–12 minutes or until cooked. Add the soy sauce for seasoning and serve sprinkled with the fresh herbs.

You can make this into a complete meal by adding noodles and/or diced vegetables to the soup. Serves 4.

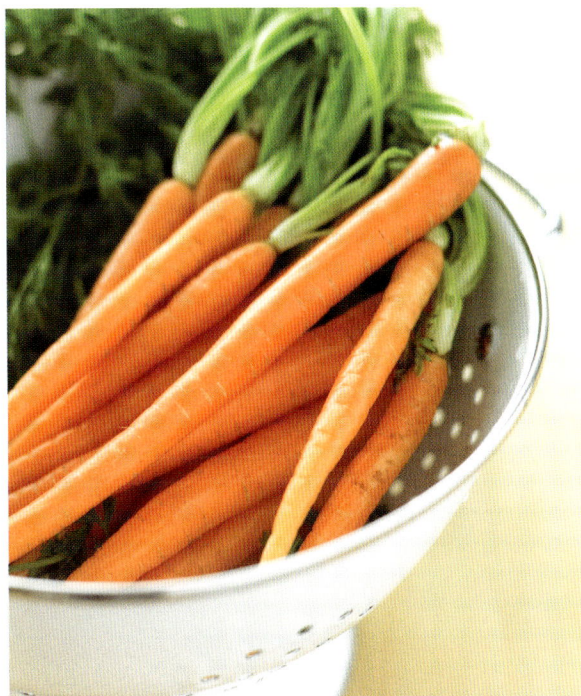

creamy parsnip soup

This is a comforting soup with a sweet nutty flavour. Parsnips are at their best in the winter months.

1 tablespoon extra-virgin olive or sesame oil
1 onion, peeled and chopped
1 clove garlic, crushed
1 teaspoon cumin seeds
600g parsnips, peeled and chopped
3 cups hot vegetable stock
1 cup milk (cow, oat, brown rice or coconut)

Heat the oil in a large saucepan and add the onion. Cook until softened and add the garlic and cumin seeds. Cook for another minute. Add the parsnips and stock and bring to the boil. Reduce the heat, cover and gently simmer for 20 minutes or until the parsnips are tender.

Cool slightly and blend using a food processor or stick blender. Add extra stock if necessary. Return to the saucepan and add the milk. Reheat and serve in warm bowls. Serves 4.

Lentils make the most fantastic and nourishing salads when combined with a delicious array of flavours such as cumin, chilli, garlic and lemon.

vegetable layers with guacamole

You'll need to wear your rubber gloves when you grate the beetroot unless you like pink hands!

1 cup mixed lettuce leaves
1 small beetroot, peeled and grated
1 carrot, grated
1 Lebanese cucumber, grated
1 zucchini, trimmed and grated
1 avocado, peeled and seeded
2 tablespoons lemon or lime juice
100g cherry tomatoes, quartered

Layer the lettuce, grated beetroot, carrot, cucumber and zucchini on two plates. Mash together the avocado and lemon or lime juice and spoon over the layered vegetables. Top with the quartered cherry tomatoes. Serves 2.

red lentil salad

This salad can also be served as an accompaniment to grilled fish, chicken or a vegetarian main course.

1 tablepoon sesame or extra-virgin olive oil
6 green onions (shallots), sliced
1 stick celery, finely chopped
2 cloves garlic, crushed
2 teaspoons cumin seeds
1/4 teaspoon dried chilli
1 cup red lentils, rinsed and drained
1 cup vegetable stock
1/4 cup lemon juice
2 tablespoons chopped dill
1/4 cup currants
soft lettuce leaves
plain yoghurt to serve

Heat the oil in a frying pan. Add the onions and celery and cook until soft. Add the garlic, cumin seeds and chilli and cook for another minute. Add the lentils and stir until well combined.

Add the vegetable stock and lemon juice and cook very gently over low to medium heat for 10–12 minutes or until all the liquid is absorbed and the lentils are tender. The lentils should still hold their shape and not be mushy.

Leave to stand for a few minutes until cool. Then fold through the chopped dill and currants. Serve in soft lettuce leaves accompanied by a dollop of plain yoghurt. Serves 4.

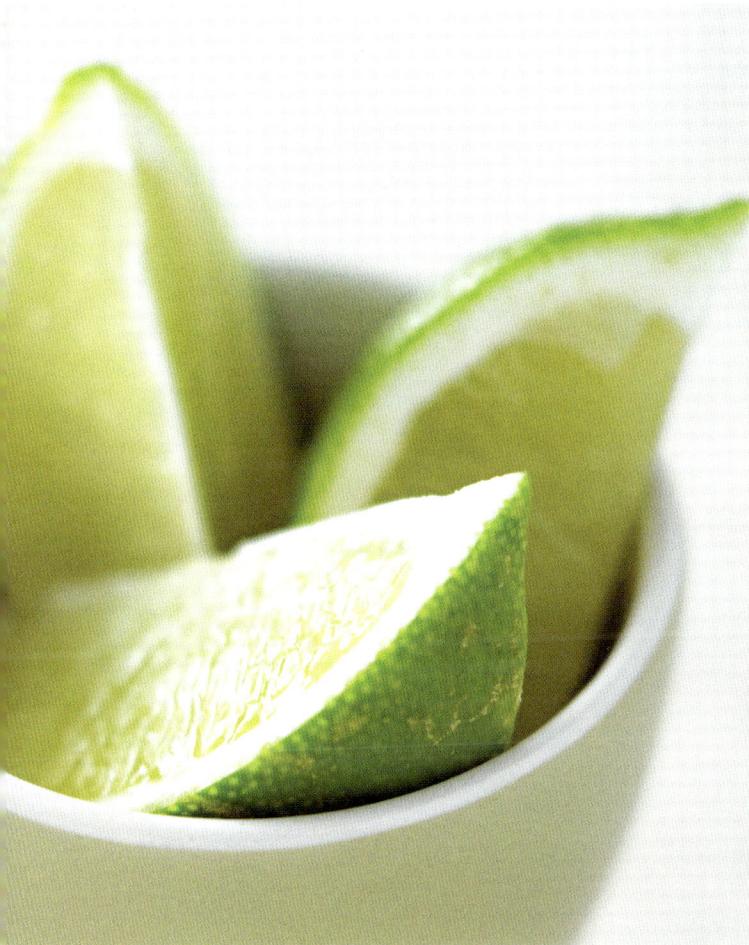

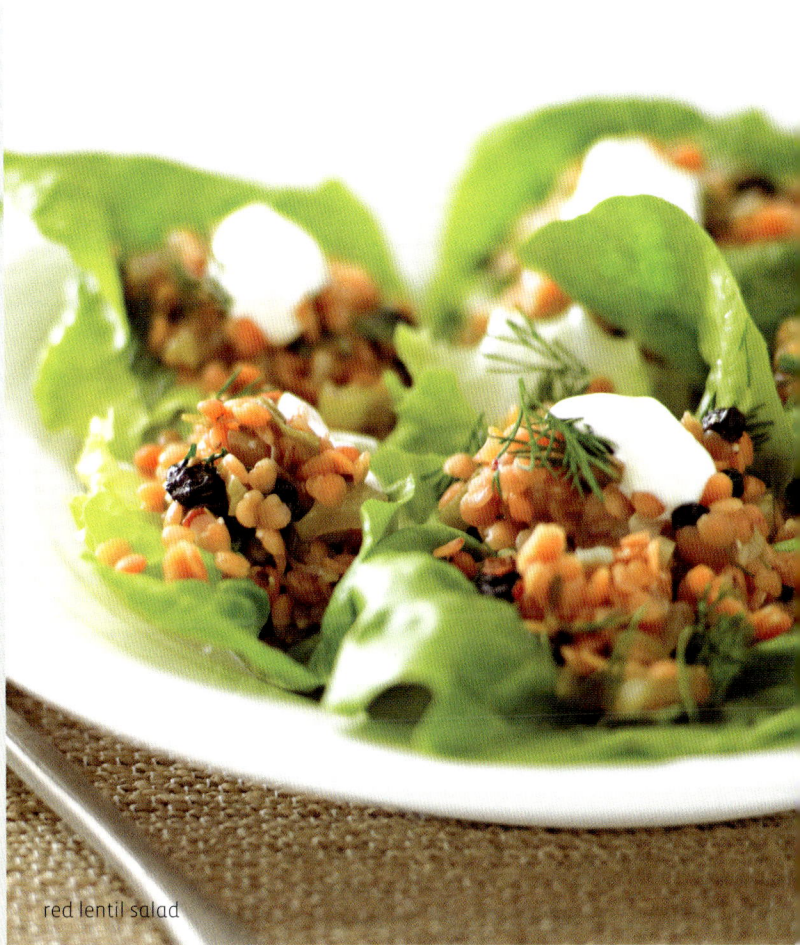

red lentil salad

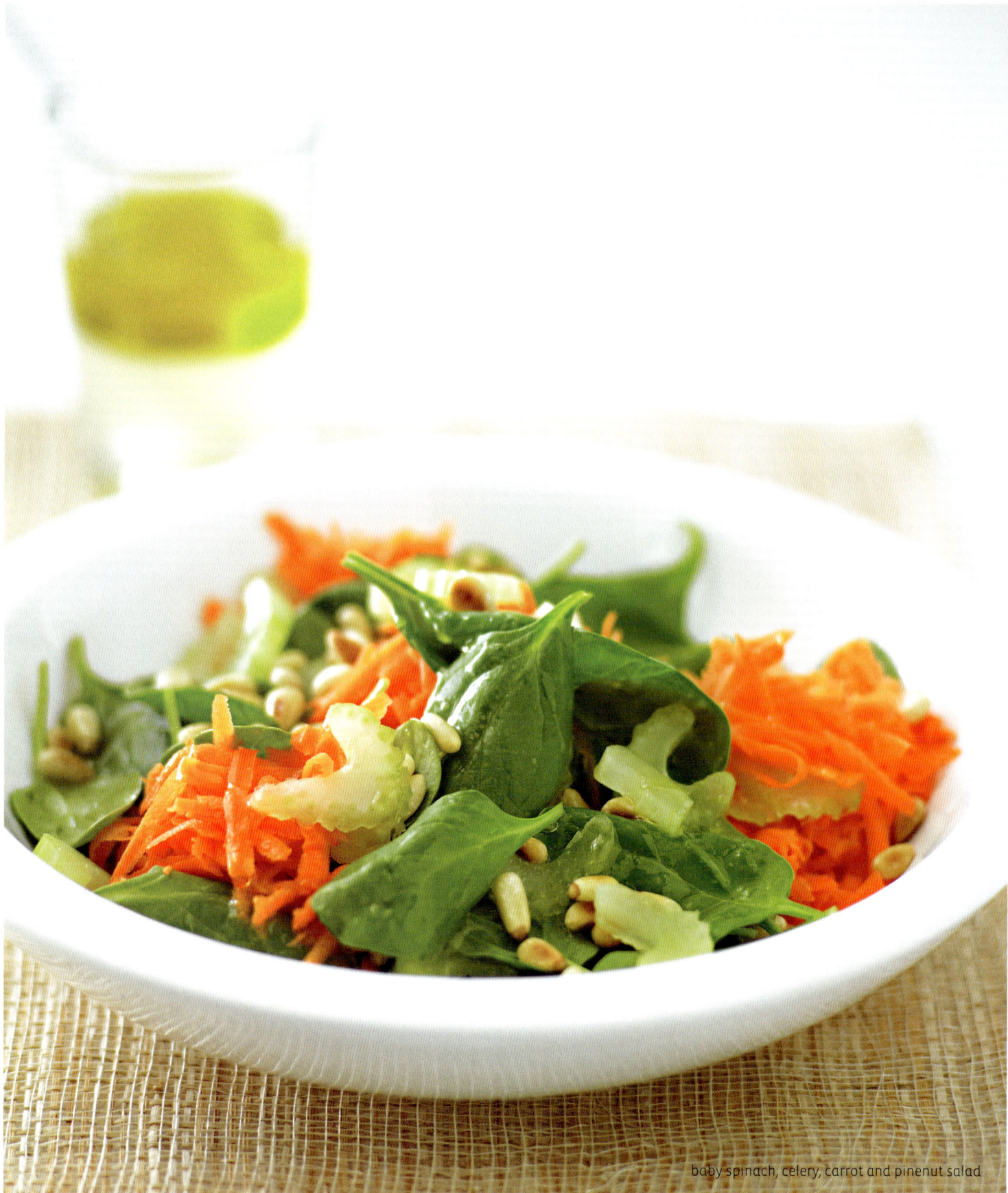

baby spinach, celery, carrot and pinenut salad

fetta and tomato tart

This simple recipe is delicious particularly with vine ripened tomatoes.

2 sheets filo pastry
extra-virgin olive oil
4 eggs
1/4 cup of milk (cow, oat or coconut)
2 sprigs fresh thyme, remove stalks
150g fetta cheese
2 tomatoes, vine ripened
sea salt and ground pepper
4 large basil leaves, shredded
2 teaspoons parsley, chopped

Preheat oven to 180ºC. Lightly grease a 20cm tart dish or two individual ramekins. Cut the two sheets of filo pastry to the size of the dish. Brush olive oil between the sheets and fit them into the dish.

Beat together the eggs, milk, thyme, sea salt and ground pepper. Crumble 100g of the fetta cheese into the beaten mixture. Pour into the tart dish and bake for 20 minutes or until set. Remove from oven and slice tomatoes. Crumble the remaining fetta, shredded basil and chopped parsley and combine with the tomato, then place on top of the tart. Serves 2.

A RAINBOW ON YOUR PLATE

Fruits and vegetables develop colour pigments to protect themselves from the damaging effects of sunlight. These colour pigments are high in health-protecting antioxidants. The deeper the pigment of fruits and vegetables, the higher the concentration of antioxidants. Red cabbage, ruby red grapefruit, kale, dark purple grapes (and to a lesser extent red grapes), orange-fleshed pumpkin, blueberries, blackberries, raspberries, strawberries — indeed, all berries — green asparagus, yellow-fleshed potatoes, watercress, spinach and all dark leafy greens are rich sources of these antioxidants. Choose a wide range of these colourful fruits and vegetables to create a rainbow on your plate.

baby spinach, celery, carrot and pinenut salad

This lovely balanced salad is enriched with toasted pine nuts.

4 cups baby spinach leaves
2 sticks celery, thinly sliced
2 carrots, thickly grated
1/3 cup pine nuts
extra-virgin olive oil and lemon juice to serve

Toss together the baby spinach, sliced celery and grated carrot and place on a serving plate. Heat a small frying pan and add the pine nuts. Cook while stirring until golden— don't leave unattended as they are easy to burn. Sprinkle the toasted pine nuts over the salad and drizzle with oil and lemon juice. Serves 4.

potato salad

You can use a mixture of extra-virgin olive oil and lemon juice or apple-cider vinegar instead of mayonnaise in this salad.

salad
800g chat potatoes
1 Spanish (red) onion, thinly sliced
1 red capsicum, seeded and thinly sliced
1 yellow capsicum, seeded and thinly sliced
200g green beans, trimmed, sliced, blanched in boiling
    water and refreshed in cold water
250g cherry tomatoes, halved
1 bunch asparagus, trimmed, sliced, blanched in boiling
    water and refreshed in cold water
2 tablespoons capers, rinsed and drained
$1/4$ cup gherkins, chopped

dressing
$1/3$ cup mayonnaise
2 tablespoons lemon juice or apple-cider vinegar
$1/4$ cup chopped chives

Place the potatoes in a large saucepan and cover with cold water. Bring to the boil and cook for 15–20 minutes or until tender. Drain, halve and leave to cool. Toss together with the other vegetables and the capers and gherkins.

Whisk together the mayonnaise and lemon juice and toss through the potato salad. Scatter with the chopped chives. Serves 6.

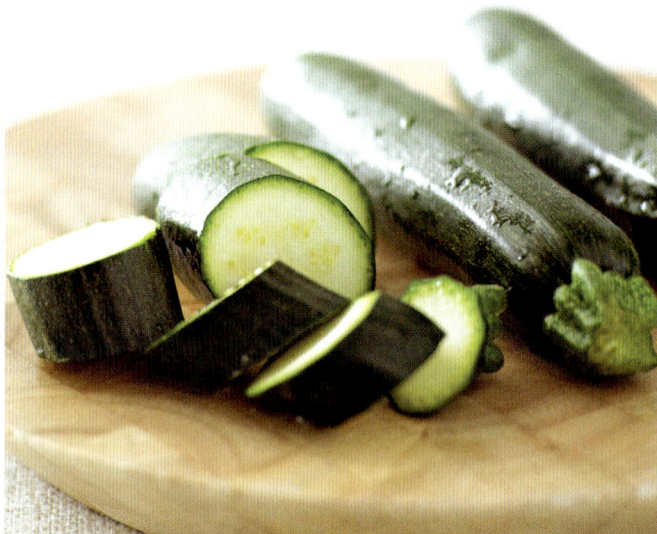

corn, zucchini and burghul salad

1 cup fine-grain burghul (cracked wheat)
3 corn cobs
3 zucchini, finely sliced
3 small red chillies, seeded and finely chopped
$1/3$ cup fresh dill, chopped
$3/4$ cup green onions (shallots), finely chopped
$1/2$ cup parsley, finely chopped
$1/3$ cup lemon juice, freshly squeezed
$1/3$ cup extra-virgin olive oil

Pour the hot water over the burghul and set aside to soak for an hour.

Blanch corn cobs in boiling water for five minutes. Drain and refresh under cold water and remove kernels from cobs. Combine with raw zucchini slices, chillies, dill, shallots and parsley.

Drain burghul and squeeze excess water out by wringing out in a clean tea-towel.

Combine the burghul with all other ingredients and let stand for an hour before serving. Serves 6.

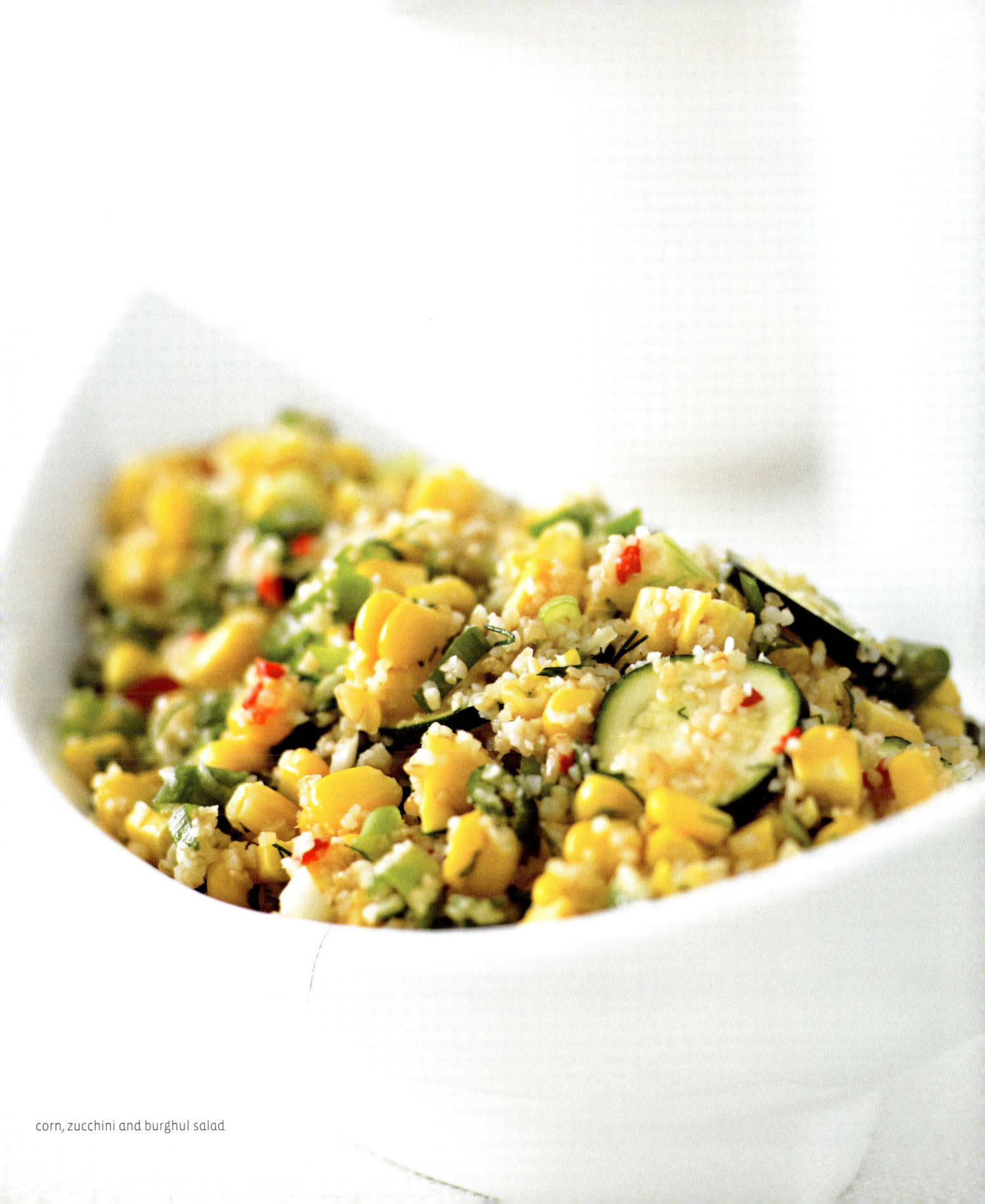

corn, zucchini and burghul salad

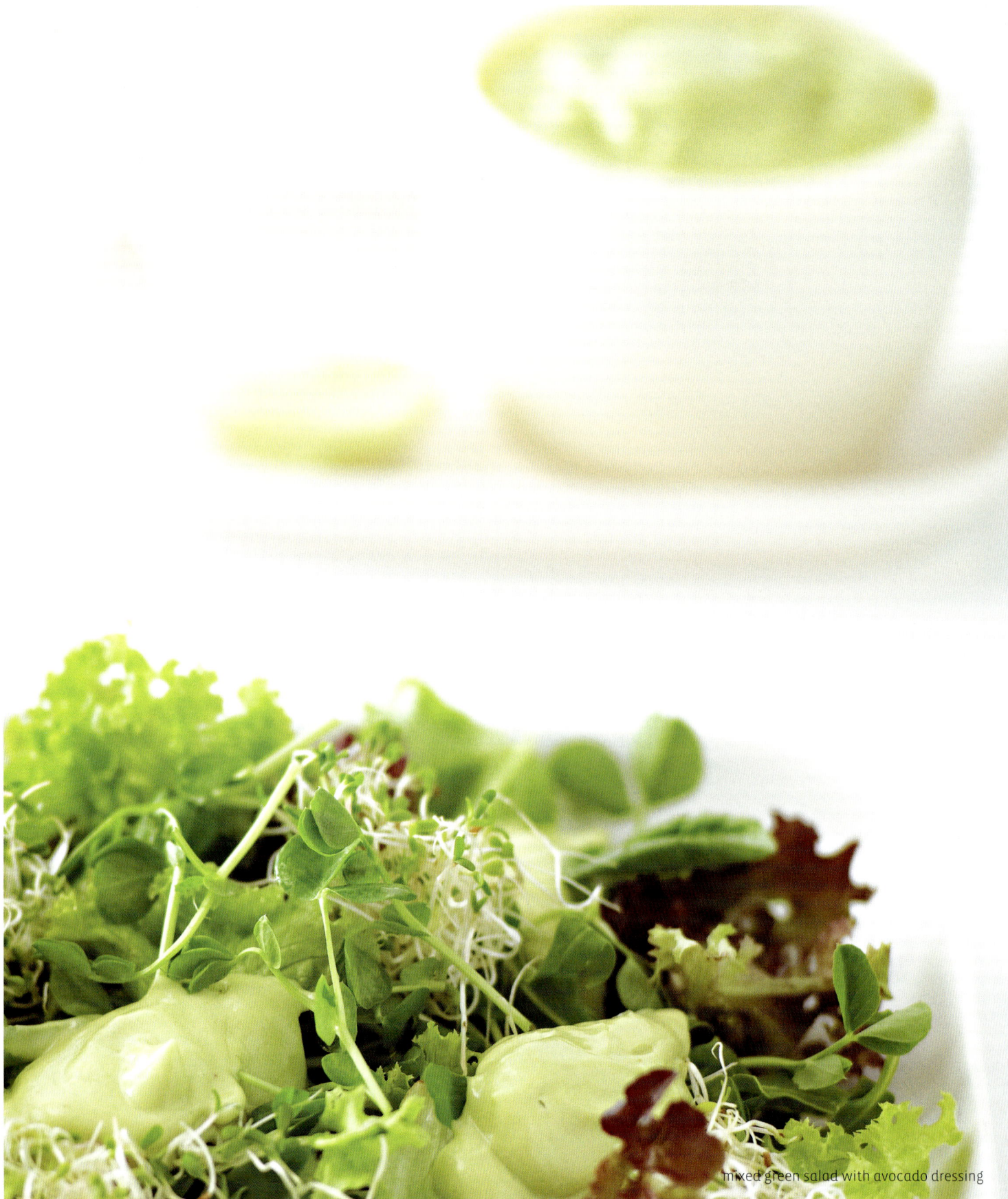

mixed green salad with avocado dressing

asparagus and snow pea salad

This crisp, crunchy and colourful salad is full of the taste of summer.

2 bunches asparagus, trimmed
500g snow peas, trimmed and halved diagonally
handful snow pea sprouts
1/2 Spanish (red) onion, thinly sliced (optional)
1/2 punnet cherry tomatoes, halved
2 tablespoons extra-virgin olive oil
1 tablespoon apple-cider vinegar
2 teaspoons lemon juice

Bring a saucepan of water to the boil and add the trimmed asparagus and snow peas. Cook for 30 seconds then drain and refresh in cold water. Pat dry with kitchen paper and toss together with the snow pea sprouts, red onion and tomatoes.

Drizzle with the oil, vinegar and lemon juice and serve. Serves 4–6.

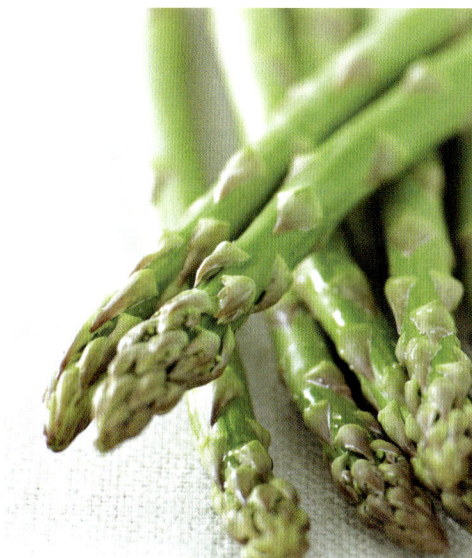

cabbage and sprout coleslaw

A new and healthy take on coleslaw using cabbage and sprouts with the juicy tang of lime and the sweetness of coconut.

salad
4 cups shredded Chinese cabbage (or regular cabbage)
1 cup grated carrot
2 cups bean sprouts, trimmed
4 green onions (shallots), thinly sliced

dressing
1/4 cup fresh lime juice
2 tablespoons sweet chilli sauce
1/3 cup coconut milk
1 teaspoon sesame oil
1/4 cup sunflower seeds

Toss together the cabbage, carrot, bean sprouts and green onion. Whisk together the lime juice, sweet chilli sauce, coconut milk and sesame oil and toss through the cabbage mixture. Pile onto a serving platter and scatter with sunflower seeds. Serves 4–6.

mixed green salad with avocado dressing

Avocados are an excellent source of nutrition and also make a delicious salad dressing.

4 cups mixed lettuce leaves
snow pea sprouts
alfalfa sprouts
1 ripe avocado
1/4 cup lemon juice
2 tablespoons plain yoghurt
1/2 teaspoon ground cumin

Toss together the lettuce and sprouts and place in a serving bowl. Place the avocado, lemon juice, yoghurt and cumin in a food processor or blender and pulse until smooth. Add water until it is of pouring consistency (about 3 tablespoons). Spoon over the salad and serve immediately. Serves 4–6.

BEANS AND LEGUMES

Think about diversifying your protein intake. Most of us know that fish, meat, poultry and dairy products are high in protein. Our bodies need protein for a variety of functions including to rebuild tissue, maintain health and assist in healing. However, many people overlook the valuable beans and legumes because they generally require some planning and preparation. It is possible to buy canned organic beans in many varieties and they can be incorporated into salads, soups, casseroles and dips. Legumes are an excellent source of protein and many are also high in calcium which helps prevent osteoporosis. Beans and legumes are the staple of many diets and they are rich in flavonoids (known anti-cancer substances) and soluble fibre.

tuna and bean salad

Tuna is an excellent source of complete protein and its minerals, trace elements and protein are not destroyed in the canning process. Choose a variety in spring water, brine or olive oil, and drain well.

150g green beans, trimmed and halved
1 cup cooked cannellini beans
1/4 Spanish (red) onion, finely chopped
10 cherry tomatoes, halved
8 kalamata olives
180g can tuna, drained
2 tablespoons extra-virgin olive oil
2 tablespoons apple-cider vinegar
2 teaspoons Dijon mustard

Blanch the green beans in a saucepan of boiling water and refresh in cold water. Combine with the cannellini beans, onion, tomatoes and olives and place on 2 plates.

Break the tuna into flakes and place on top of the salad. Whisk together the oil, vinegar and mustard and drizzle over the salad. Serves 2.

chickpea and tabouli salad

This dish is brimming with vitamin C and calcium and tastes wonderful. If you don't like spicy food, you can leave out the pepper and mixed spice.

1 cup dried chickpeas, soaked overnight in cold water
2 bunches flat-leaf parsley
1 bunch mint
4 large ripe tomatoes, diced
2 Lebanese cucumbers, diced
1/2 teaspoon ground black pepper
1 teaspoon mixed spice
2–3 tablespoons extra-virgin olive oil
1 lemon, juiced
sea salt

Drain the water from the soaked chickpeas and rinse well. Place the chickpeas in a saucepan and cover with cold water. Bring to the boil and reduce the heat. Simmer for about 45 minutes or until the chickpeas are tender. Drain and cool.

Trim the stalks from the parsley and mint and roughly chop the leaves. Combine with the diced tomato, cucumber, pepper and mixed spice (if using). Fold through the cooked chickpeas and toss through the olive oil and lemon juice. Season with a little sea salt. Serves 4.

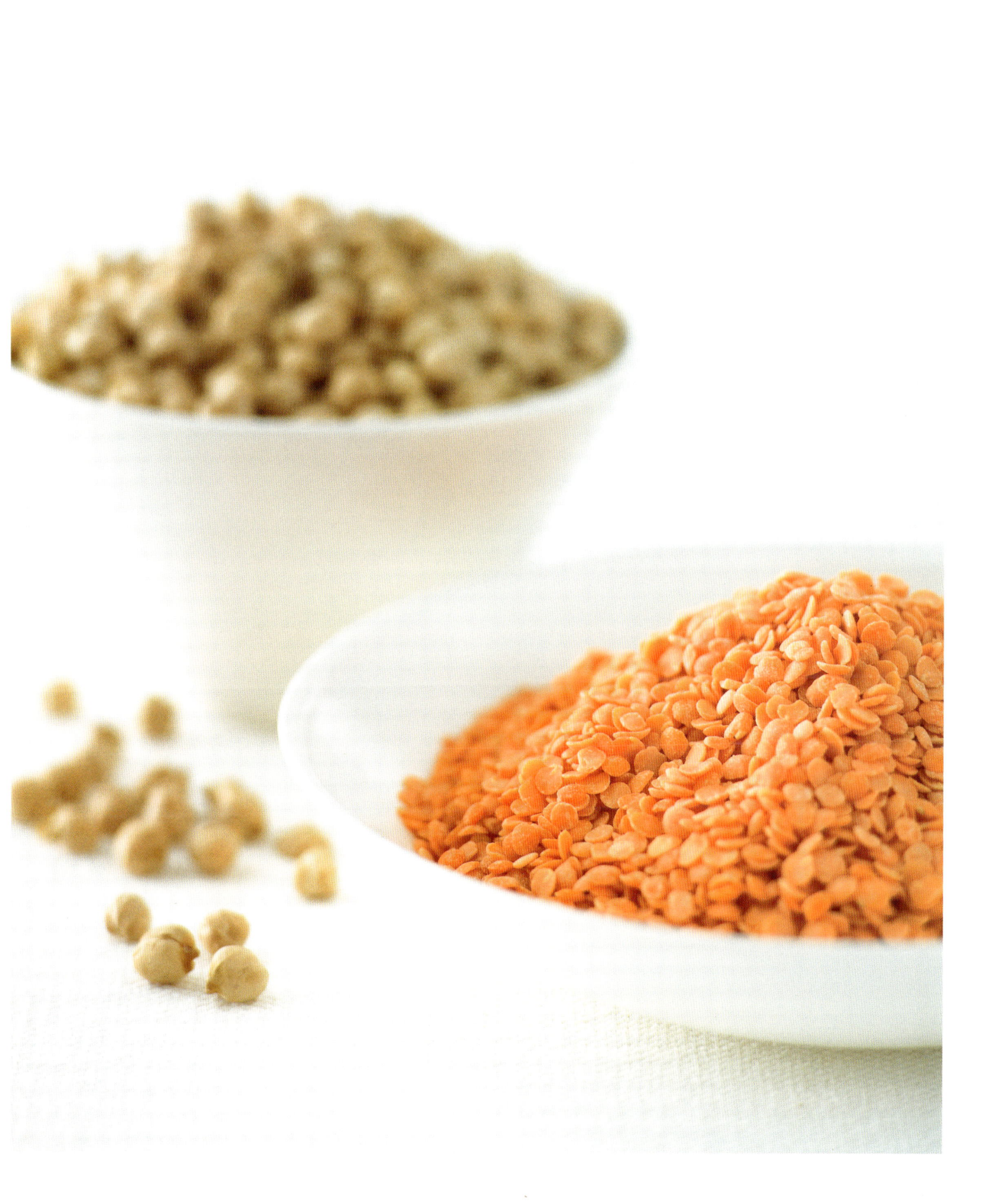

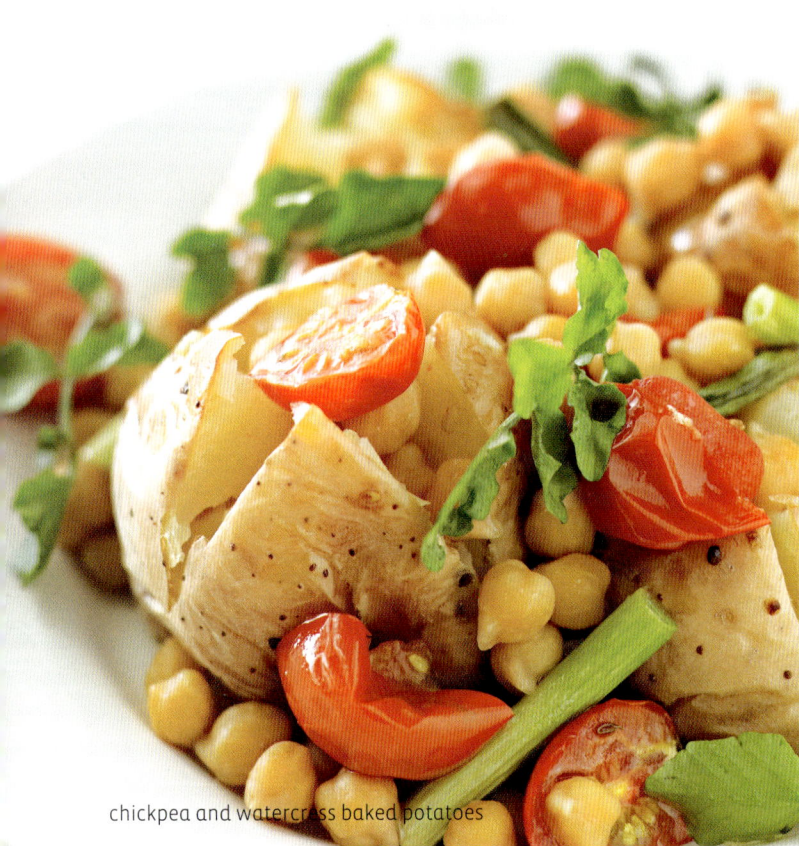

chickpea and watercress baked potatoes

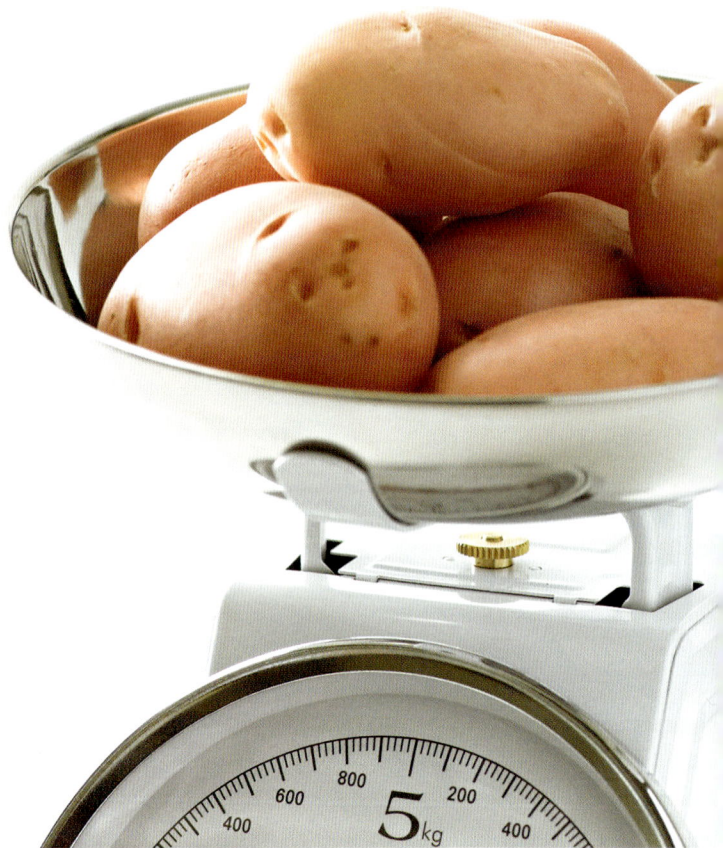

chickpea and watercress baked potatoes

Watercress is often forgotten, but is very flavoursome with its slightly bitter flavour. It is also high in antioxidants and calcium.

4 medium potatoes
125g cherry tomatoes, halved
4 green onions (shallots), cut into 4cm lengths
2 teaspoons extra-virgin olive oil
1 clove garlic, crushed
$1/4$ teaspoon cumin seeds
2 cups cooked chickpeas, warmed
1 cup watercress, trimmed into bite-size pieces
1 tablespoon white-wine vinegar

Heat the oven to 190°C. Wash and dry the potatoes and pierce with a fork. Place on a baking tray in the oven and cook for 1 hour or until tender.

Toss the cherry tomatoes and green onions with olive oil and garlic and place on a baking tray lined with baking paper. Sprinkle with cumin seeds. Add to the oven for the last 15 minutes of the potatoes' cooking time.

Remove the tomato mixture from the oven and toss together with the watercress, chickpeas and vinegar. Make cross-cuts in the top of the potatoes and open. Fill with the warm chickpea salad. Serves 4.

Potatoes baked in their jackets make a great light meal, full of goodness and fibre. They are easy to grow, and many varieties are available for the home gardener.

salmon and tzatziki baked potatoes

This is another delicious idea for a jacket potato filling.

4 medium potatoes
2x210g cans red salmon, drained
2 green onions (shallots), finely sliced
$1/3$ cup plain yoghurt
$1/2$ Lebanese cucumber
1 small clove garlic, crushed (optional)
1 tablespoon chopped mint
dill to serve

Heat the oven to 190°C. Wash and dry the potatoes and pierce with a fork. Place in the oven and cook for 1 hour or until tender.

To make the tzatziki, grate the cucumber and place in a sieve. Gently squeeze out the excess liquid. Stir the cucumber into the yoghurt and fold through the garlic (if using) and mint.

Gently combine the red salmon with the sliced onions. Make cross-cuts in the top of the potatoes and open. Fill with the salmon mixture and top with a tablespoon of tzatziki and a sprinkling of dill. Serves 4.

rainbow couscous

500ml chicken stock, preferably homemade (see page 57)
2 tablespoons lemon infused virgin olive oil
$1/2$ teaspoon ground allspice
$1/2$ teaspoon ground cumin
$1/2$ teaspoon ground coriander
1 teaspoon caraway seeds
2 small red chillies, deseeded and finely chopped (optional)
1 lemon, juiced and 2 teaspoons zest
600g couscous
1 medium Spanish (red) onion, chopped
$1/2$ green capsicum, chopped
$1/2$ red capsicum, chopped
2 corn cobs, blanched for five minutes, refreshed in cold water and kernels removed
1 cup fresh peas, blanched for five minutes, refreshed in cold water
1 cup macadamia nuts, roasted and coarsely chopped
$1/3$ cup fresh coriander, chopped
$1/3$ cup fresh parsley, chopped
sea salt and black pepper

Combine chicken stock, oil, spices, chillies, juice and zest in a saucepan and bring to the boil. Pour over couscous in a large bowl. Stir with a fork to separate the grains. Add onion, capsicums, corn kernels, peas, nuts and herbs and season with ground sea salt and black pepper. Serves 6.

rice pilaf

$1^1/2$ tablespoons mustard seed oil
2 teaspoons mustard seeds
2 teaspoons cardamom seeds
2 teaspoons cumin seeds
8 whole cloves
5 green onions (shallots), chopped into 1cm pieces
6 cloves garlic, crushed
2 cinnamon sticks
200g button mushrooms
3 cups basmati rice
1 medium red capsicum, chopped
1 medium green capsicum, chopped
3 carrots, sliced and quartered
250g cauliflower florets
150g broccoli florets
4 cups chicken stock
$1^1/2$ cups of fresh peas

Heat mustard seed oil in a large, deep frying pan. When hot, stir in mustard, cardamom and cumin seeds and cloves and stir until they start to pop. Add green onions, garlic and cinnamon and cook, stirring often, until green onions begin to soften. Add mushrooms and a little more oil if necessary and stir to combine. Mix in the rice and stir to coat with the oil mixture. Add all the remaining ingredients except for the peas and stir to combine. Cover tightly and cook over low heat for 15 minutes. Add the peas, recover and cook for another 5 minutes. Separate the grains with a fork and serve. Serves 6–8.

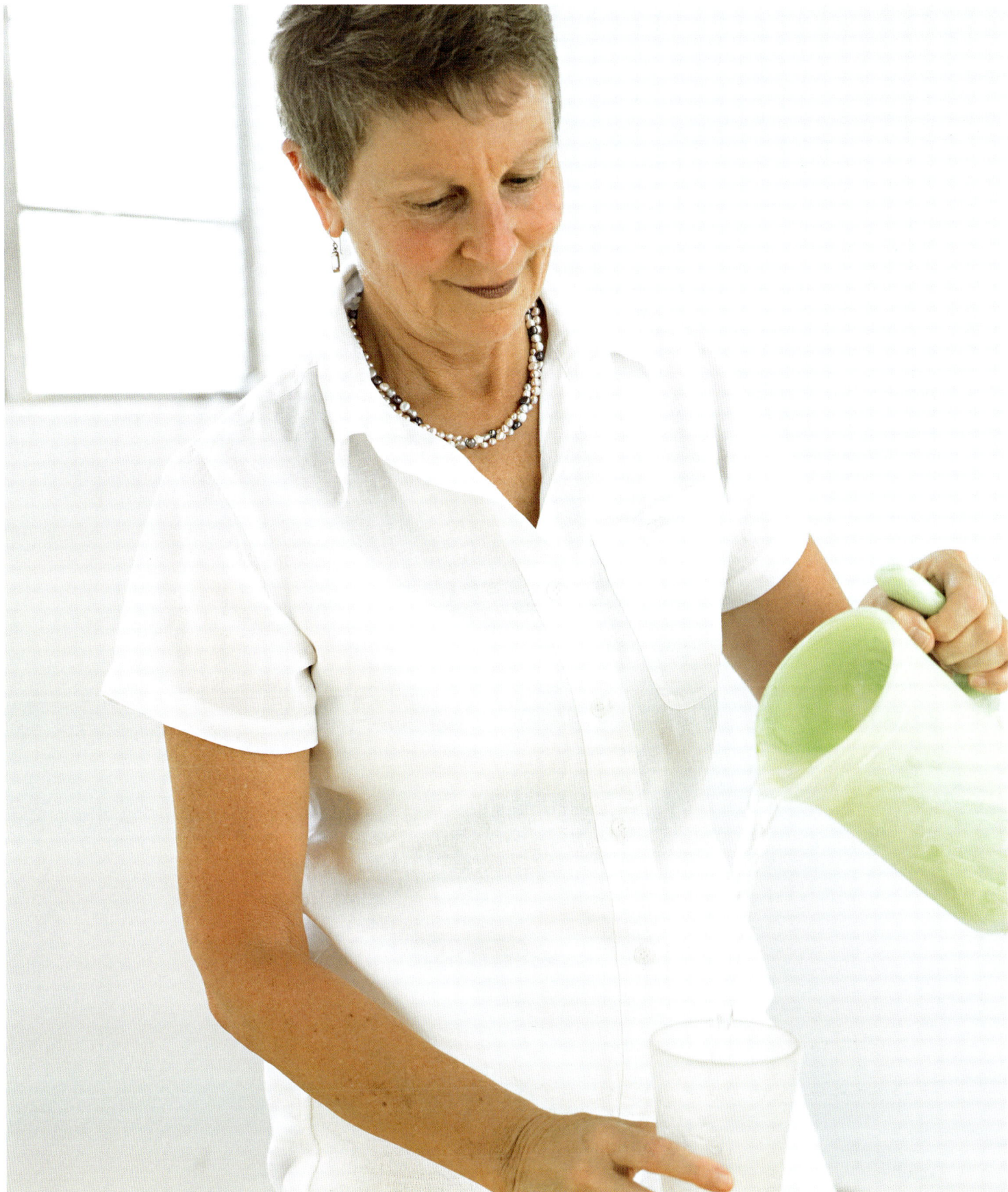

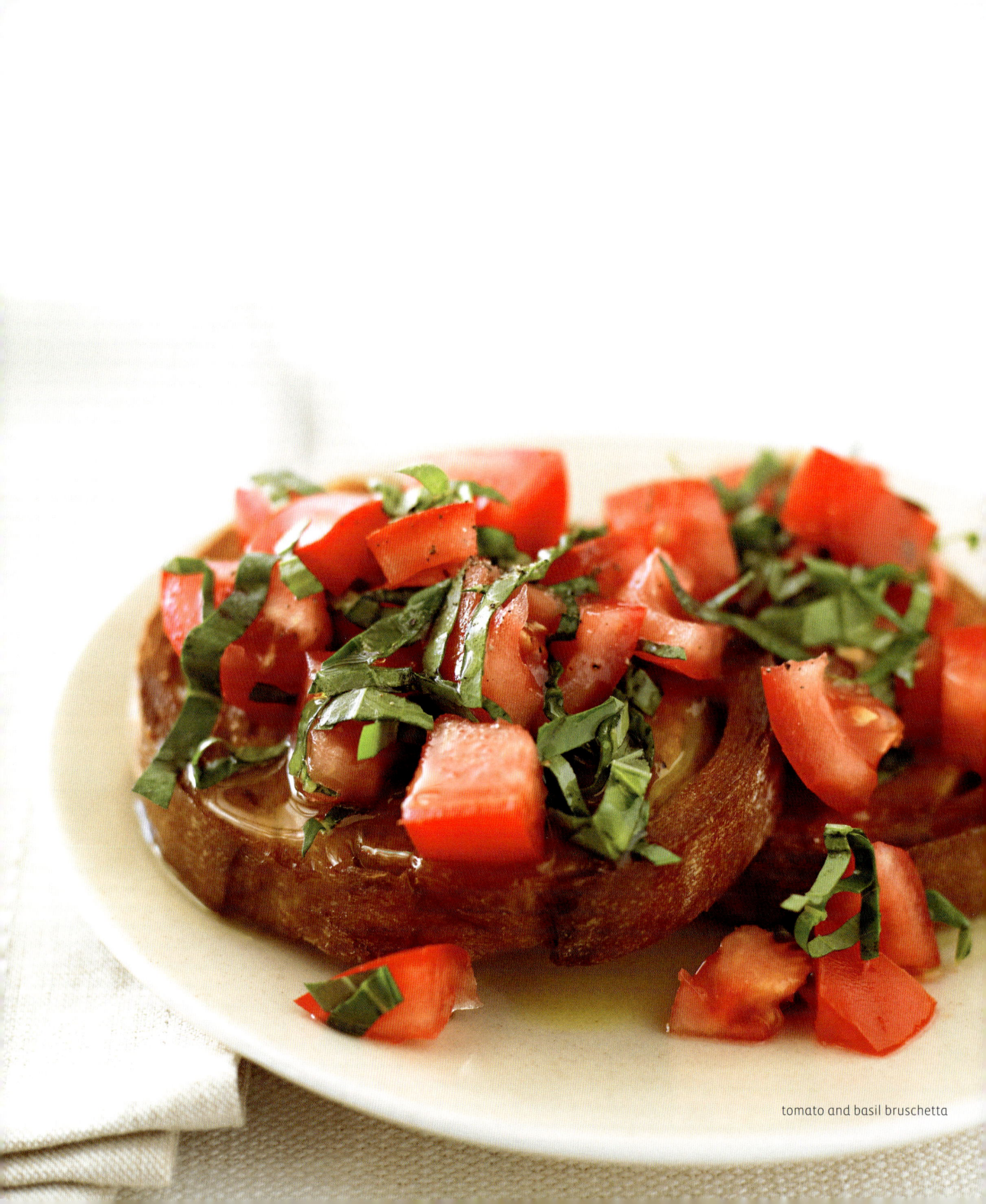

tomato and basil bruschetta

beetroot jam

This can be eaten with bread, as a dip with raw vegetables or added to jacket potatoes or other baked vegies. It will keep in the refrigerator for up to two weeks.

1kg beetroot, peeled and grated
2 medium onions, thinly sliced
2 cups freshly squeezed orange or ruby red grapefruit juice
1 cup apple concentrate or 1 cup brown sugar
3/4 cup apple-cider vinegar
2 cinnamon sticks

Place all ingredients in a saucepan and simmer for 45 minutes, stirring occasionally. When most of the moisture has evaporated, remove from the heat and allow to cool. Store in clean glass bottles and refrigerate.

tomato and basil bruschetta

You will need a chargrill pan or barbecue to make this. Without the tomato topping it is a wonderful version of garlic bread.

4 vine-ripened tomatoes
1 tablespoon chopped fresh basil
8 slices sourdough bread
2 tablespoons extra-virgin olive oil
1 clove garlic, peeled

Heat the grill pan or barbecue until very hot. While it is heating, dice the tomatoes and stir through the chopped basil.

Cook bread on both sides until golden and crispy and brown around the edges. Place on a serving platter and rub each slice of bruschetta with the peeled clove of garlic. (The harder you rub the more garlicky it will taste.) Drizzle with oil and spoon over the tomato and basil. Serves 4.

HERBS AND SPICES

Many culinary herbs and spices have a long history as medicines and more than 50 per cent of all modern drugs are based on the active ingredients found in plant material. Herbs and spices are often very high in antioxidants, vitamins, trace minerals, volatile oils and antibacterial qualities. And some spices and herbs, like cinnamon, cloves, turmeric and bay leaves have been shown to increase the activity of insulin. Peppermint has long been used as an aid to digestion as its volatile oils stimulate the appetite and the production of bile. Anise, which tastes a little like liquorice, has been used for flatulence. Ginger is one of the most ancient therapeutic herbs and is used as an antibacterial, blood thinner or anticoagulant and anti-nausea herb.

toasted spinach, tomato and cheese sandwiches

If you don't have any ricotta, then use all cheddar (you will only need about 3/4 of a cup). These flatbread toasted sandwiches also taste fabulous filled with leftover roasted vegetables.

1/4 cup finely chopped Spanish (red) onion
3 cups baby spinach leaves
pinch grated nutmeg
1/2 cup grated cheddar cheese
1/2 cup ricotta cheese
2 Lebanese breads, halved and split open
2–3 tablespoons tomato paste
extra-virgin olive oil

Heat up a toasted sandwich maker. In a bowl, combine the onion, spinach, nutmeg and cheeses. Open the halves of Lebanese bread and spread with the tomato paste. Fill with the spinach mixture. Brush each side of the bread with a little oil and place in the sandwich maker for 2–3 minutes or until golden, crisp and the filling is cooked. Serves 2.

SALT

Natural crystal salt is essential to life and has been mined or harvested for thousands of years. However, modern methods of mining and chemical treatments have reduced salt into a damaging substance called sodium chloride. Natural crystal salt consists of not just sodium and chloride but contains all the same 84 elements that are present in the human body and can be used in moderation in cooking and at the table.

chicken salad wraps

4 sheets lavash or mountain bread
1/2 cup hommus (see page 97)
11/3 cups shredded cooked chicken
2 cups mixed soft lettuce leaves
1 cup alfalfa sprouts
4 cherry tomatoes, quartered
2 cups shredded carrot
1 tablespoon tamari or soy sauce
1/3 cup sweet chilli sauce

Place the sheets of bread on a clean work surface and spread with the hommus. Divide the chicken, lettuce, sprouts, tomatoes and carrot into 4 and place on the sheets of bread.

Combine the tamari and sweet chilli sauce and drizzle over the chicken salad. Roll up each wrap, cut into 2 and serve. If not serving immediately then wrap in cling wrap. Serves 4.

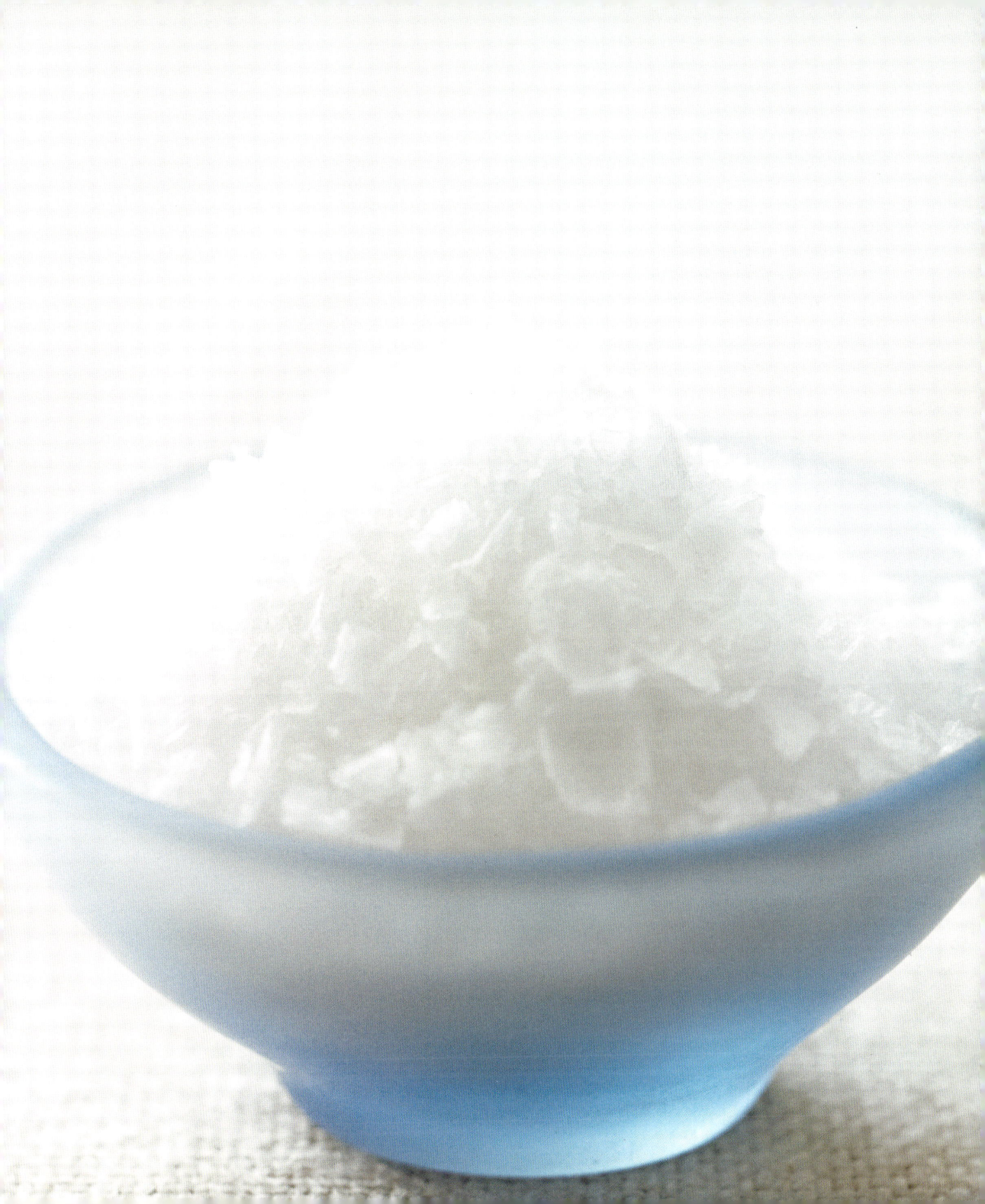

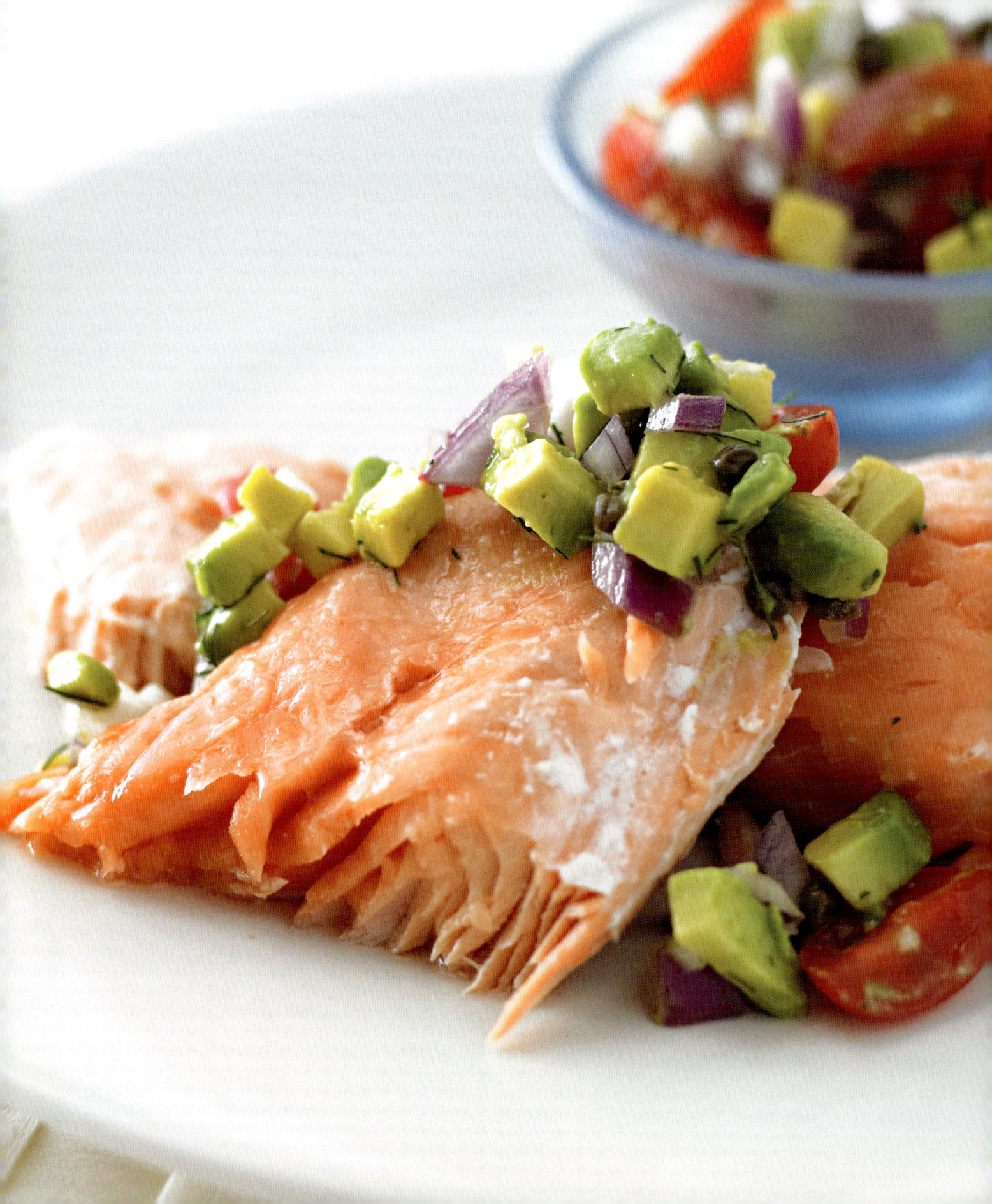

Main
Meals

main meals

Making the decision to eat a wholesome diet doesn't mean you have to spend hours in the kitchen preparing complicated dishes or compromise on flavour.

BY USING GOOD quality ingredients you can create meals which are both delicious and satisfying, and the following easy-to-prepare meals will appeal to the whole family.

At the Quest for Life Centre our main meals include plenty of raw and cooked vegetables as well as fish or organic chicken. Our chef Doug cooks with seasonal, fresh produce and avoids using processed foods or foods with artificial colours, preservatives and flavours. His platters of delicious salads, vegetables and other foods appeal to our guests even if they have a jaded appetite. Many people are astounded at how good our 'healthy' food tastes.

We include protein in our main meals. Protein is essential for good health, as all repair and rebuilding of cells in the body is dependent on it and people who adopt a low-protein diet often become weary and lethargic. Protein foods are divided into two types: complete and incomplete. Complete proteins contain the eight essential amino acids and these are necessary for growth and cell repair. Complete proteins can be found in meat, fish, eggs and dairy products. Incomplete proteins are found in the vegetable kingdom and contain some of the essential amino acids, but not all. In addition to vegetables, they are in legumes, beans, seeds, nuts, whole grains and lentils. If you are a vegetarian you need to combine your incomplete proteins to ensure you get a healthy intake of all essential amino acids. Eating plenty of seeds, brown rice, nuts and legumes as well as vegetables is a good way to do this.

We don't serve red meat at the Quest for Life Centre as we believe it is not essential in our diet. However, listen to your body. If you have a strong craving for red meat you may well need some of its nutrients. Restricting your intake to once or twice a week will satisfy your nutritional needs and choosing lean, organic, paddock-raised lamb or beef with all excess fat removed is best.

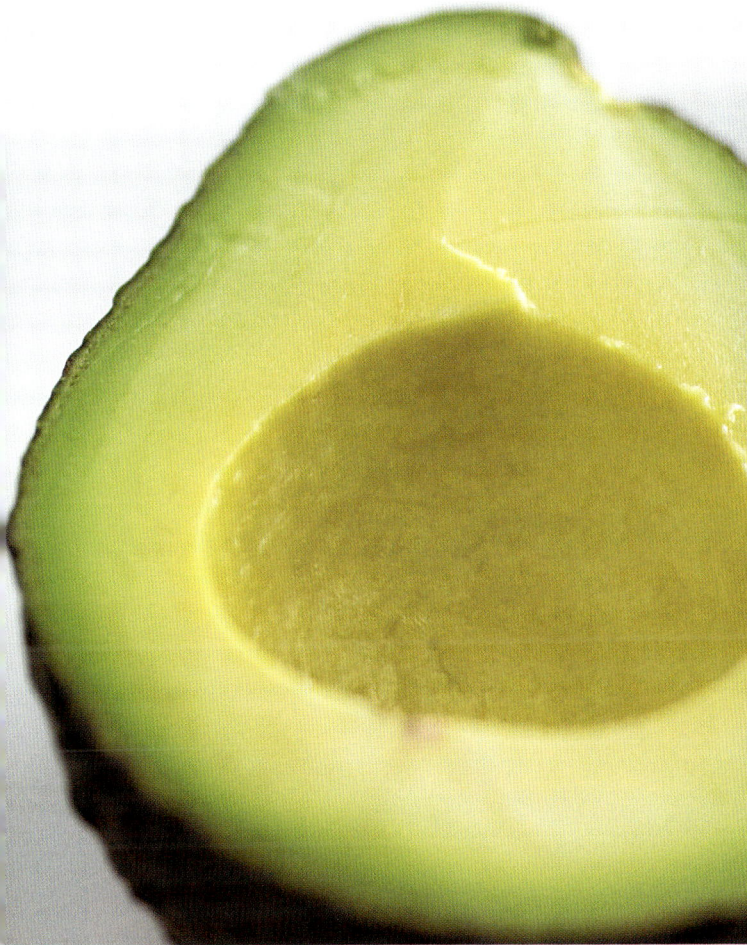
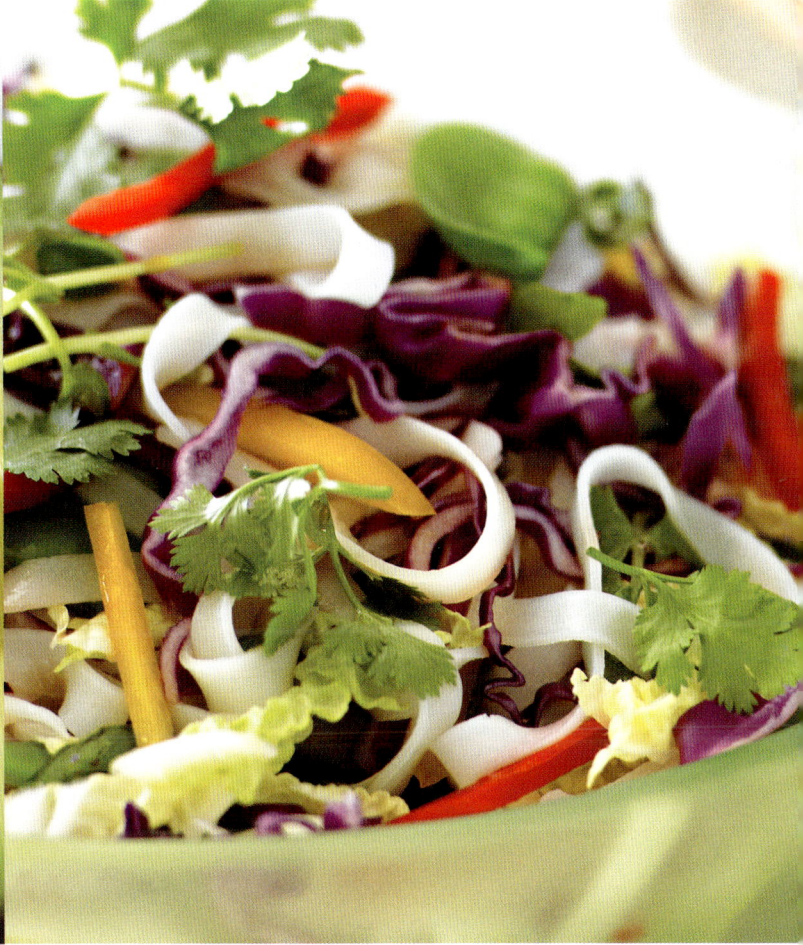

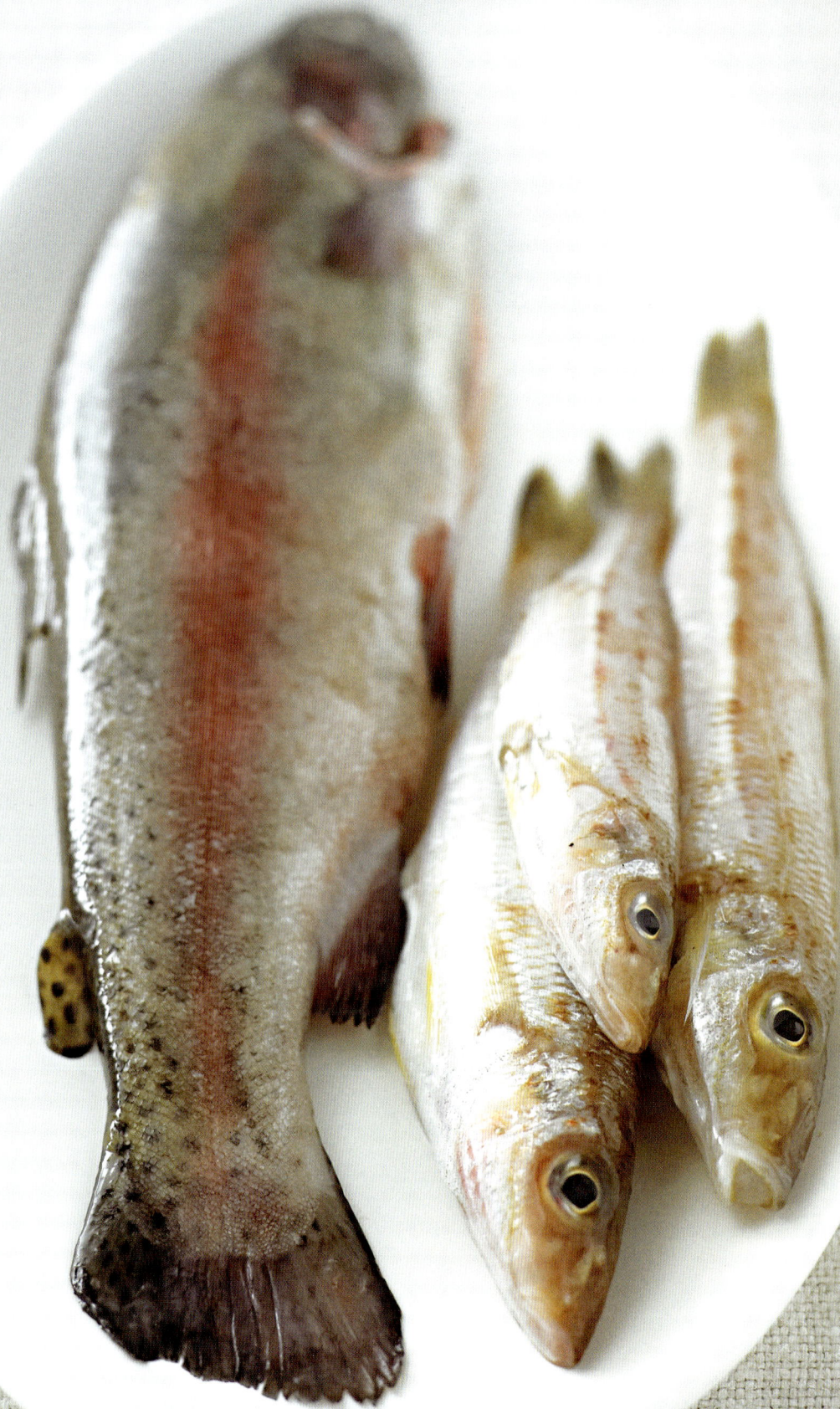

baked fish and vegetables

You can add another couple of fish fillets to this recipe without increasing the quantity of the sauce.

1 tablespoon extra-virgin olive oil
1 leek, finely chopped
1 red capsicum, seeded and finely diced
2 cloves garlic, crushed
100g mushrooms, chopped
400g can chopped tomatoes
1/4 cup chopped parsley
2 bunches asparagus, trimmed or snow pea sprouts
4x200g fillets deep-sea white-fleshed fish (perch, ling etc.)

Preheat the oven to 200°C. Heat the oil in a large frying pan and add the leek and capsicum. Cook over a medium heat until soft. Add the garlic, mushrooms and tomatoes and simmer for 10 minutes.

Place the fish fillets in a large baking dish and bake in the oven for 5 minutes while the vegetables are cooking. Remove from the oven and spoon over the vegetable mixture. Return to the oven and cook for 15–20 minutes or until the fish is cooked through.

Steam the asparagus and place on top of the cooked fish with chopped parsley or garnish with snow pea sprouts. Serves 4.

steamed fish with greens and miso dressing

The miso dressing in this recipe gives the greens a great flavour. Couscous or brown or basmati rice is a delicious accompaniment to this dish.

2 tablespoons chopped coriander
grated rind of 1 lemon
sea salt and black pepper
2x200g firm white deep-sea fish fillets (perch, ling etc.)
4 cups assorted green vegetables
   (broccoli, bok choy, snow peas etc.),
   trimmed and cut into bite-size pieces
2 tablespoons bean or snow pea sprouts
1 tablespoon sweet white miso
1 tablespoon tahini
2 tablespoons tamari or soy sauce
1 tablespoon lemon juice

Combine the coriander, lemon rind, salt and black pepper. Gently press mixture onto the top side of each fish fillet. Place in a steamer and cook for 7–10 minutes or until the fish is opaque and cooked. Steam or blanch the vegetables.

While the fish and vegetables are cooking, place the miso, tahini and tamari in a bowl. Whisk dressing together with 1 tablespoon of lemon juice and 1 tablespoon of water until smooth.

Place the vegetables on two plates. Top with the fish and drizzle with the dressing. Scatter with bean or snow pea sprouts. Serves 2.

crab and water chestnut spring rolls

You can also use prawn or chicken mince to make these spring rolls—frying the mince along with the ginger, garlic and celery. Serve these spring rolls with a simple green salad with an Asian-flavoured dressing for a lovely main meal.

3 teaspoons sesame oil
1 large onion, finely chopped
2 cloves garlic, crushed
1 tablespoon grated ginger
2 tablespoons tamari or soy sauce
1 cup grated carrot
1 cup bean sprouts
235g can water chestnuts, drained and finely chopped
1 cup finely shredded Chinese cabbage
300g fresh crab meat
18 sheets 20x20cm square spring roll pastry
1 egg white, lightly beaten
1/3 cup sweet chilli sauce

Preheat oven to 220˚C. Heat the sesame oil in a large frying pan and add the onion. Cook until soft and add the garlic and ginger. Cook for another minute then stir through the tamari or soy sauce.

Remove from the heat and stir through the carrot, bean sprouts, water chestnuts, cabbage and crab.

Place one sheet of the pastry on a flat surface. Place 1/3 cup of the mixture in one corner of the pastry sheet and fold the bottom corner over the filling. Fold in the sides and continue to roll up firmly. Place on a baking tray and repeat with the remaining mixture. Brush with the egg white and bake in the oven for 20 minutes or until golden. Serve with the sweet chilli sauce for dipping. Serves 4–6.

panfried fish with roast beetroot

Beetroot is one of the most brightly coloured vegetables and is packed with anti-oxidants that promote good health. It retains its nutrients even when cooked.

4 medium beetroots, peeled and cut into wedges
1 Spanish (red) onion, cut into wedges
1 tablespoon extra-virgin olive oil
1 teaspoon cumin seeds
1 teaspoon sea salt
4x200g fish fillets
1 teaspoon extra-virgin olive oil, extra
2 lemons, cut into wedges
1/2 bunch watercress or salad of bitter leaves

Heat the oven to 200˚C. Toss the wedges of beetroot and onion in the olive oil and sprinkle with the cumin seeds and sea salt. Place in a single layer on a baking tray. Cook for 45 minutes or until tender.

Heat a large frying pan and brush the fish fillets with the extra oil. Cook for 2 minutes on each side or until opaque and cooked through. Serve with the beetroot and onion, and some lemon wedges. Accompany with watercress or a bitter leaf green salad. Serves 4.

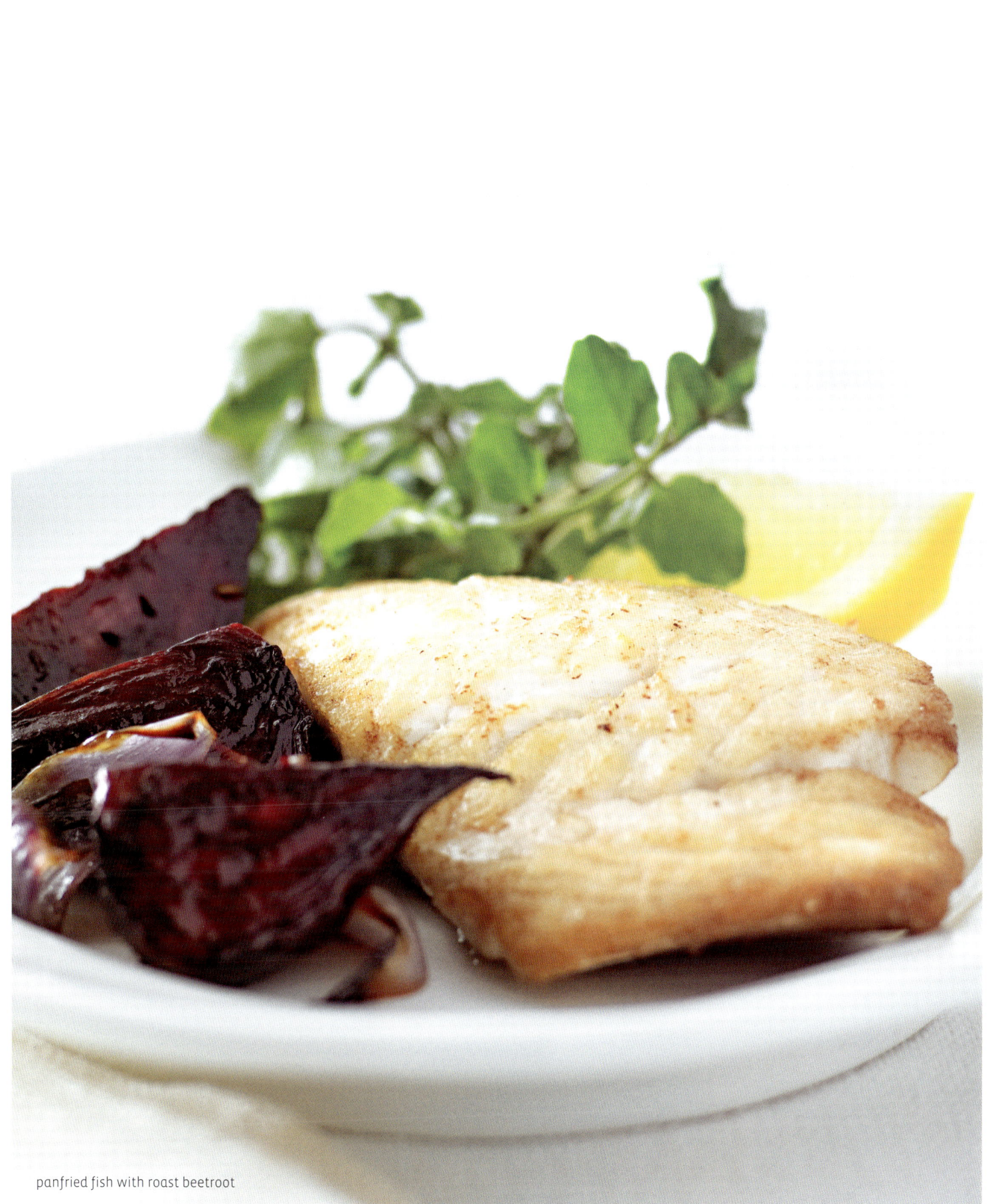

panfried fish with roast beetroot

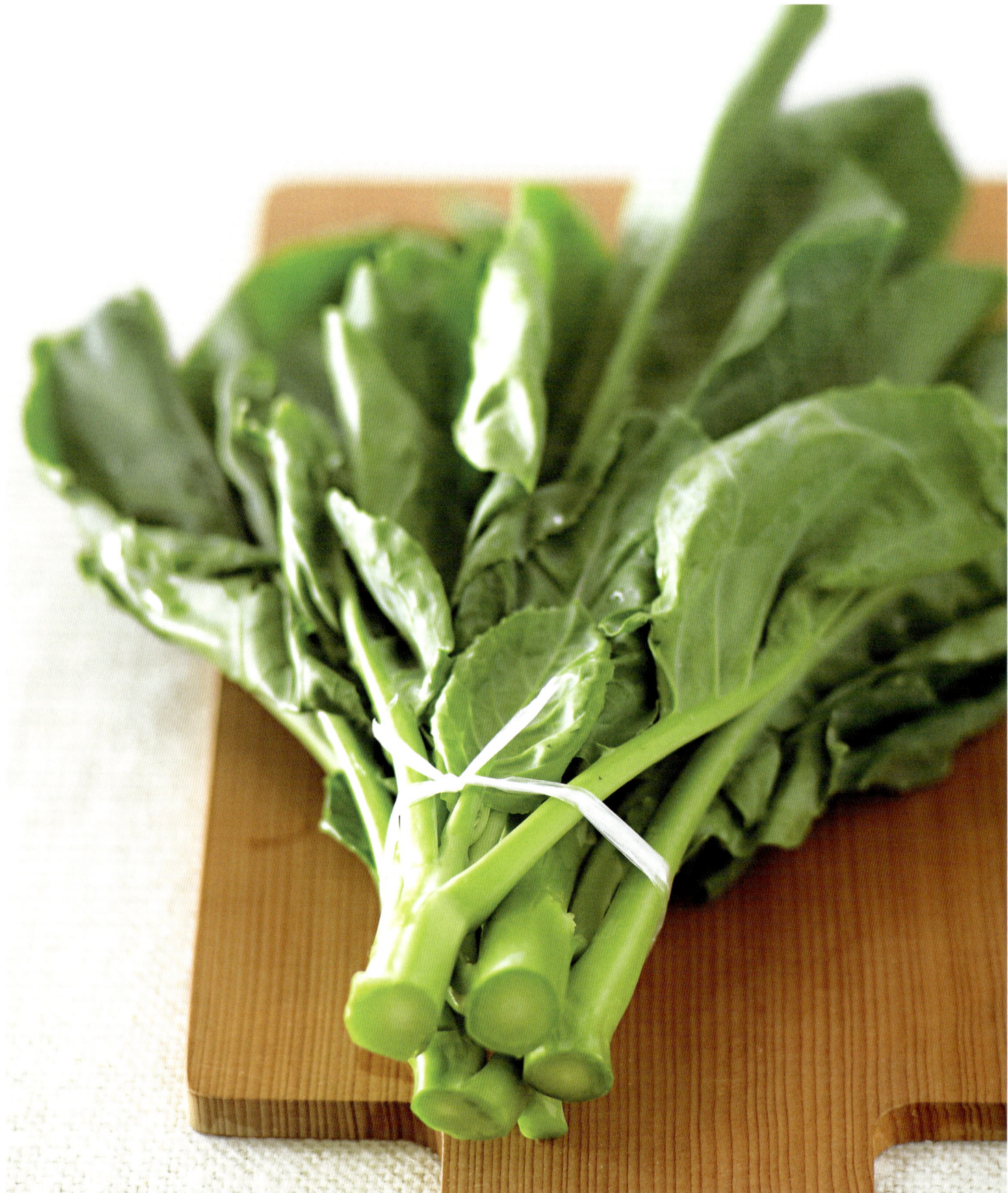

grilled lemon calamari

The younger and smaller the calamari, the more tender the finished dish will be.

750g small calamari
3 tablespoons extra-virgin olive oil
1 lemon, zest and juice
pinch dried chilli flakes (optional)
wedges of lemon to serve

Clean the calamari and turn the body inside out. Slice into 1cm rings and cut the tentacles and fins into bite-size pieces.

Combine the olive oil, lemon zest and juice. Preheat the grill or barbecue until very hot. Grill the calamari for 5 minutes or until it turns white and is brown around the edges. Scatter with the dried chilli flakes (if using) and serve with wedges of lemon and steamed rice or a rocket salad. Serves 4.

soy and sesame salmon with chinese greens

To toast sesame seeds heat a small frying pan and simply add the sesame seeds. Cook while stirring and tossing for a minute or so or until golden. Don't take your eyes off them as they can burn quickly.

4 salmon fillets
1 tablespoon honey
2 tablespoons soy sauce or tamari
2 teaspoons sesame oil
1 teaspoon five-spice powder
1 teaspoon ground cumin
1 tablespoon sesame seeds, lightly toasted
400g assorted Chinese green vegetables
   (gai lum, bok choy etc.), trimmed
2 tablespoons oyster sauce
wedges of lemon

Place the salmon fillets in a shallow dish. Combine the honey, soy sauce or tamari and sesame oil and pour over the salmon. Cover and marinate for 30 minutes.

Preheat the grill or barbecue. Sprinkle the salmon with the five-spice powder and ground cumin and cook for 4–5 minutes on each side.

Steam the Chinese vegetables until tender and toss with the oyster sauce. Place the vegetables on 4 plates and top with the salmon fillets. Sprinkle with the sesame seeds and serve with wedges of lemon. Serves 4.

Salmon always looks spectacular, but is also spectacularly easy to prepare. Choose wild salmon from the less polluted southern oceans whenever possible.

barbecued fish parcels with dill

This is a real favourite at the Centre. It's so simple to prepare, looks great and the nutrition is sealed in.

4 salmon fillets
1 tablespoon unsalted butter, sesame oil or
  extra-virgin olive oil
1/3 cup chopped dill
4 green onions (shallots), finely sliced
8 mushrooms, finely sliced

Place each salmon fillet on a sheet of foil. Top each piece of salmon with 1 teaspoon of butter or oil and one quarter of the dill, green onions and mushrooms. Loosely fold the foil around the fish to make a well-sealed parcel.

Heat the barbecue to medium and cook the parcels for 15 minutes or until the salmon is cooked through. Alternatively, bake in the oven at 180°C for 12 minutes.

Serve with a selection of salads and baked potatoes or wholegrain bread. Serves 4.

baked salmon with cherry tomato and avocado salsa

You can serve this hot or cold and it's delicious accompanied by steamed new potatoes and a green salad.

2kg whole salmon
1 lemon, sliced
750g cherry tomatoes, quartered
1 small Spanish (red) onion, finely chopped
2 avocados, diced
1/3 cup dill, chopped
1/4 cup capers, rinsed (optional)
sea salt

Preheat the oven to 180°C. Place 2 large sheets of baking paper on a flat baking tray. Place the salmon on top of the baking paper and place the lemon slices in the cavity. Loosely wrap the salmon in the baking paper, sealing the edges well so completely enclosed. Cook in the oven for 30–40 minutes and let stand for 10 minutes before serving. When ready to serve, carefully remove the skin from the top side of the salmon and place the fish on a large platter.

For the salsa, combine the tomatoes, onion, avocado, dill and capers. Season with sea salt and spoon over the salmon. Serves 8.

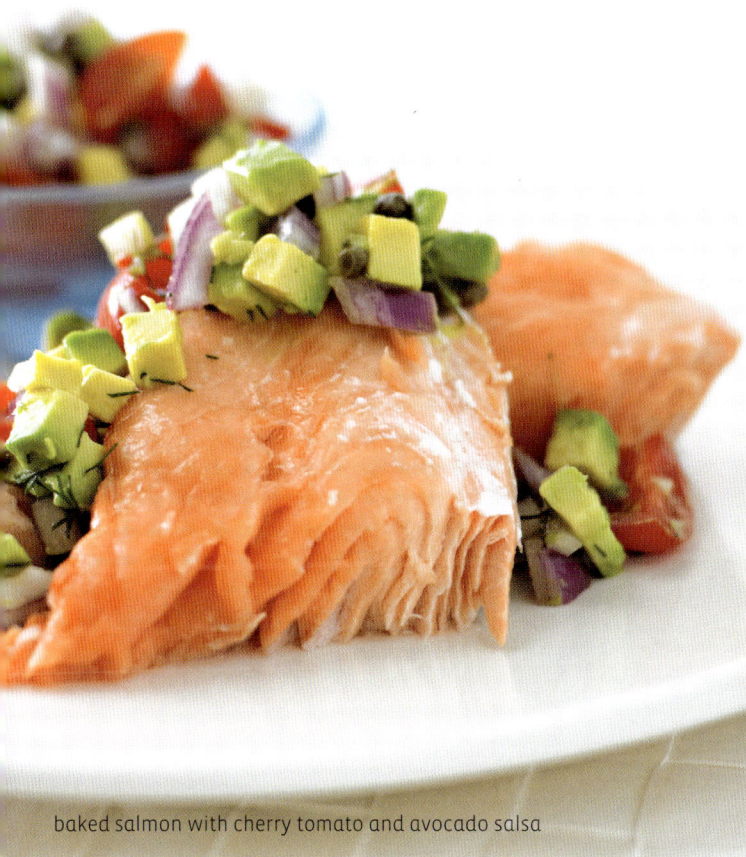

baked salmon with cherry tomato and avocado salsa

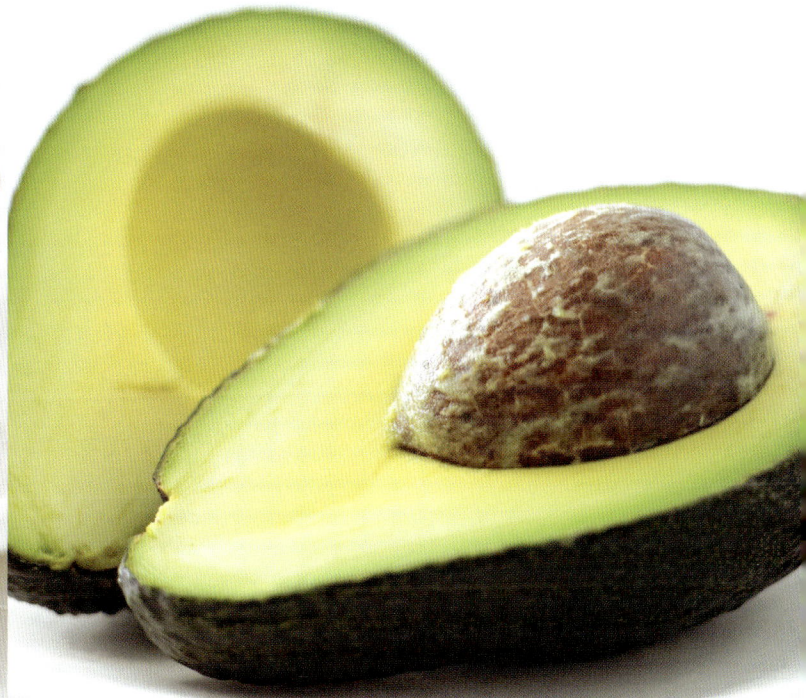

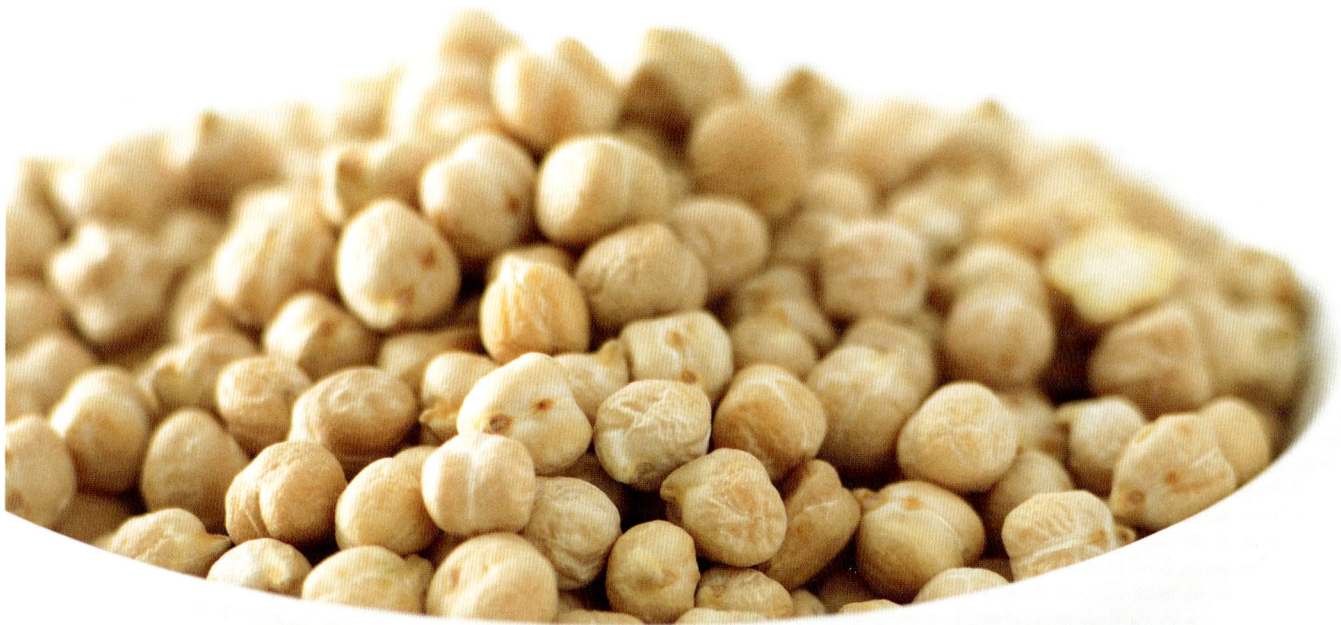

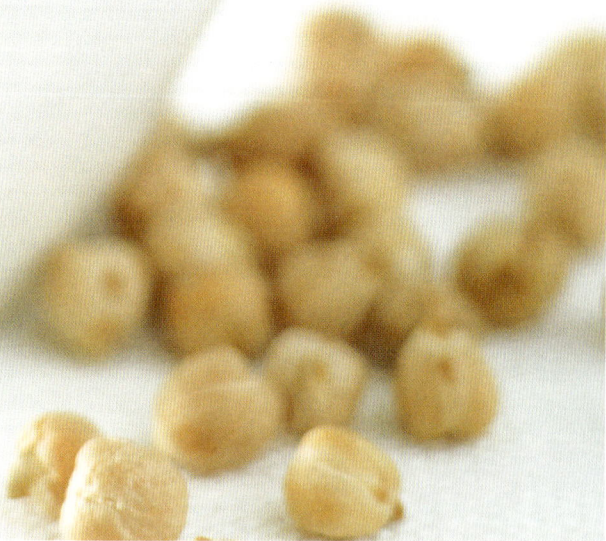

barbecued fish and vegetables with chickpeas

A lovely way to serve this dish is to pile the food on large white platters and place in the middle of the table. Everyone can help themselves and the meal will have a wonderful casual feel.

1/3 cup extra-virgin olive oil
1 lemon, juiced
1 tablespoon Dijon mustard
1 teaspoon raw sugar
1/2 cup chopped mixed fresh herbs
   (parsley, chives, mint, basil etc.)
sea salt and black pepper
2 kumara (orange sweet potatoes), peeled and sliced
2 red capsicums, seeded and cut into strips
2 green capsicums, seeded and cut into strips
1 eggplant, sliced
4 zucchinis, sliced lengthways
3 bunches asparagus, trimmed
2 cups cooked chickpeas
1–2 tablespoons extra-virgin olive oil, extra
8 fillets firm fish (blue-eye cod, salmon, snapper, tuna etc.)
wedges of lemon to serve

Whisk together the extra-virgin olive oil, lemon juice, mustard, sugar and herbs. Season to taste with sea salt and black pepper and reserve.

Heat the barbecue and toss the vegetables in half the olive oil. Barbecue in batches until golden and cooked. Remember to start with the kumara as that will take longest to cook. Place the cooked vegetables on a large platter, scatter over the chickpeas and drizzle over the dressing.

Coat the fish fillets in the remaining oil and barbecue for 4–5 minutes (turning once), or until cooked through and opaque. Place on a separate platter. Serve with wedges of lemon and crusty wholemeal rolls. Serves 8.

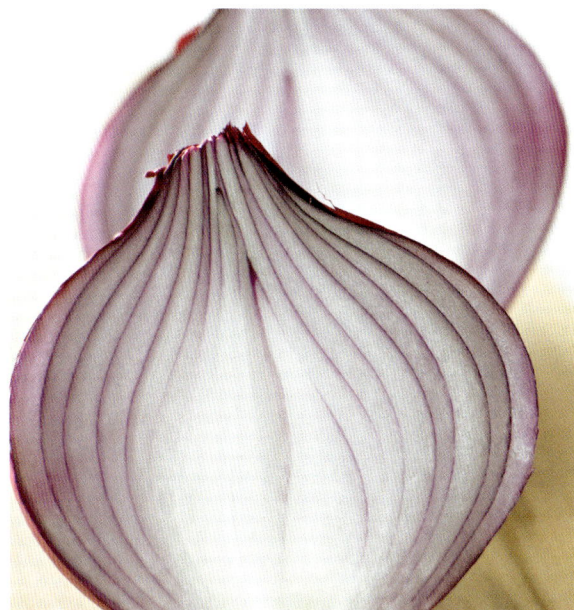

prawn and chickpea salad

Prawns and chickpeas might not seem an obvious combination but it works! Smoked trout is a delicious alternative to the prawns.

750g cooked prawns, peeled and deveined,
   or 2 smoked trout, skin and bones removed
1/2 Spanish (red) onion, finely chopped
1 clove garlic, crushed
1 small head fennel or 3 sticks celery, finely diced
250g cherry tomatoes, halved
500g cooked chickpeas
1/3 cup lemon juice
1/3 cup extra-virgin olive oil
1/2 cup torn basil leaves
1/2 cup chopped flat-leaf parsley
sea salt and black pepper

Combine the prawns or trout, chickpeas, onion, garlic, fennel and cherry tomatoes in a large bowl. Whisk together the lemon juice, oil, basil and parsley. Drizzle over the salad and season with sea salt and black pepper. Serve with crusty sourdough bread and a rocket salad. Serves 4–6.

ginger and star anise chicken

Star anise adds a most exquisite flavour to this dish. It is also one of the most beautiful-looking spices. You'll find star anise and Chinese rice wine at an Asian supermarket.

1 large chicken
1/2 cup soy sauce or tamari
1 cup Chinese rice wine
1 1/2 cups chicken stock
4 star anise
2 tablespoons sliced ginger
2 cloves garlic, squashed
4 green onions (shallots)
1/4 cup brown sugar
500g pumpkin, peeled and cubed
steamed rice and Asian green vegetables to serve

Remove any fat and the skin of the chicken. Place chicken in a saucepan and add the other ingredients (except pumpkin). Bring to the boil, reduce heat and cover tightly. Simmer for 25 minutes, then add the pumpkin and simmer for another 20 minutes. Turn off the heat and let stand for 15 minutes.

Carefully lift the chicken out of the cooking liquid and carve into 8 pieces. Place on a platter along with the cubes of pumpkin and spoon over a little of the cooking liquid. Serve with steamed rice and Asian green vegetables. Serves 4.

CANCER AND FOOD

Research indicates that the foods we eat can influence our susceptibility to certain types of cancer. High energy and high-fat diets, which can lead to obesity, increase the risk of some cancers, while we know that 90 per cent of all human-made chemicals, many of which appear in processed foods or are used in the production of food, are carcinogenic. Plant-based diets high in fresh fruits, vegetables, legumes and whole grains can help to prevent cancer.

grilled chicken with sugar-snap pea and spinach salad

8 chicken thigh fillets
4 roma tomatoes, halved lengthways
200g sugar-snap peas, blanched
3 green onions (shallots), finely chopped
100g baby spinach leaves
2 tablespoons extra-virgin olive oil
1 tablespoon apple-cider vinegar

Heat the barbecue or grill and cook the chicken thighs for 5 minutes on each side or until golden and cooked through. Cover with a sheet of foil and keep warm while you make the salad.

Grill the tomatoes for 2 minutes until just soft. Combine the sugar-snap peas, green onions and baby spinach leaves and place in a serving dish. Place the grilled tomatoes in the salad. Drizzle salad with extra-virgin olive oil and apple-cider vinegar and serve with the grilled chicken. Serves 4.

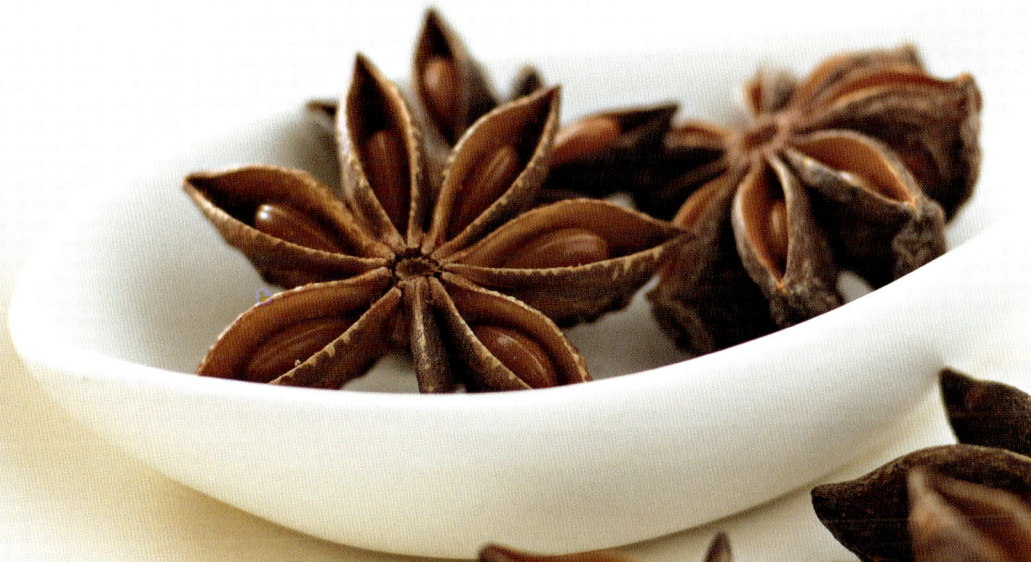

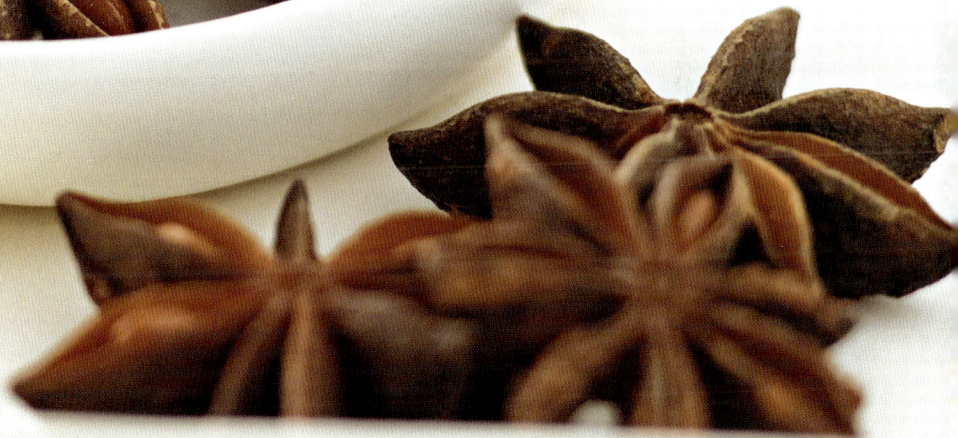

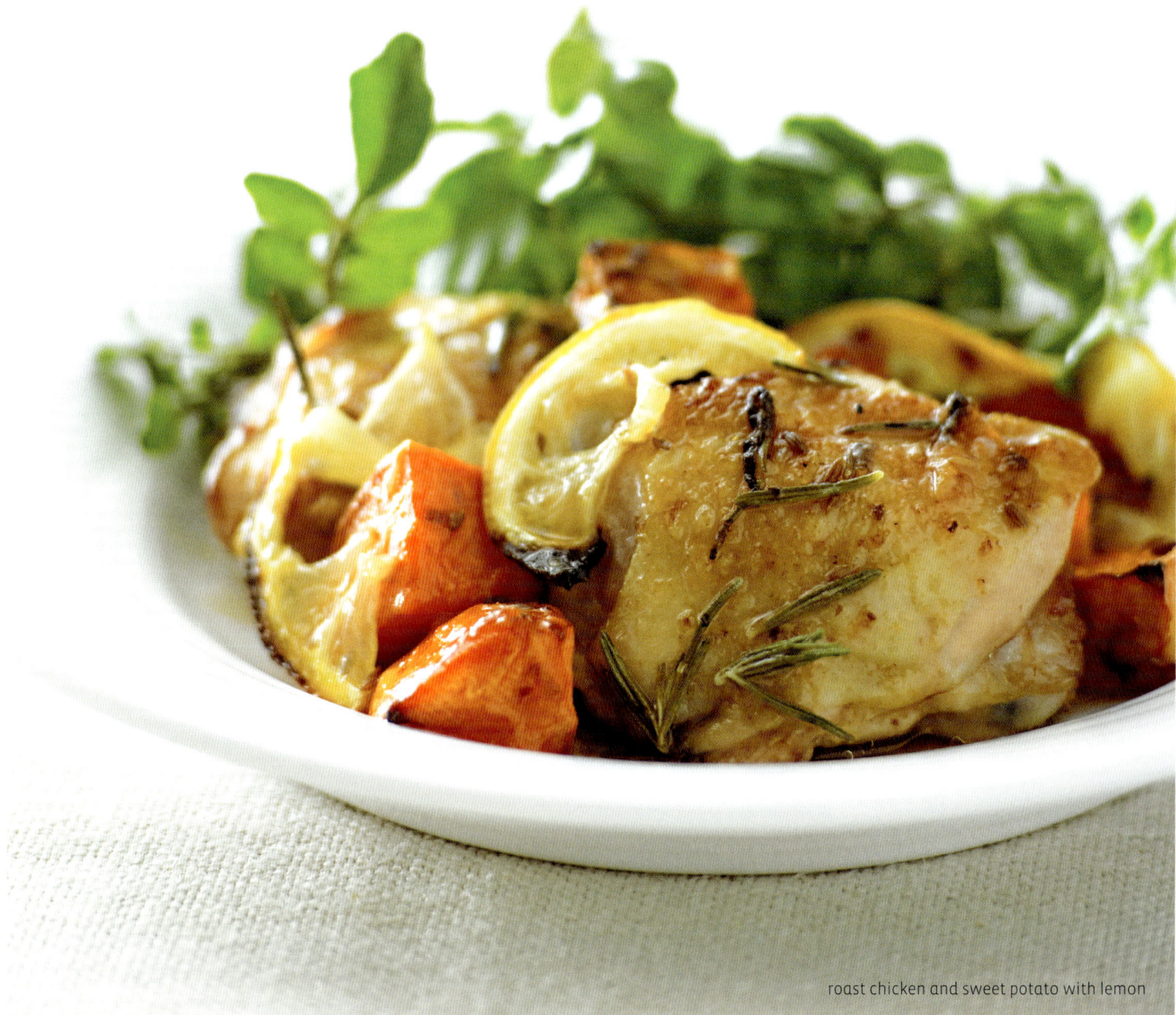

roast chicken and sweet potato with lemon

roast lemon chicken with white bean puree

The aroma of this roast chicken wafting through the house will sharpen everyone's appetite. Lemon-infused extra-virgin olive oil is delicious and makes this dish sublime. It's available at delicatessens and some supermarkets.

1 large chicken, washed and patted dry with a paper towel then rubbed with 1 teaspoon extra-virgin olive oil (lemon-infused if possible)
small bunch fresh thyme
1 lemon, cut into quarters
2 cups cooked cannellini beans
2 tablespoons extra-virgin olive oil (lemon-infused if possible)
1 clove garlic, crushed
1 teaspoon cumin seeds, lightly toasted
2 tablespoons lemon juice
sea salt and black pepper
1 cup baby rocket leaves

Preheat the oven to 220°C. Put the lemon and thyme into the chicken's cavity and place on a rack in a roasting pan above water. Roast in the oven for 80 minutes. Top up water under the roasting chicken from time to time and baste the chicken with the juices.

While the chicken is cooking, place the beans, garlic, cumin seeds and lemon juice in a food processor and blend until smooth. Warm in a small saucepan and stir through the oil. Season with sea salt and black pepper.

Remove the chicken from the oven, loosely cover with foil and a clean tea towel and leave to rest for 10 minutes before carving. Carve the chicken and drizzle with some of the cooking juices left in the roasting pan. Spoon the white bean puree onto 4 plates, top with the chicken and scatter over the baby rocket leaves. Serves 4.

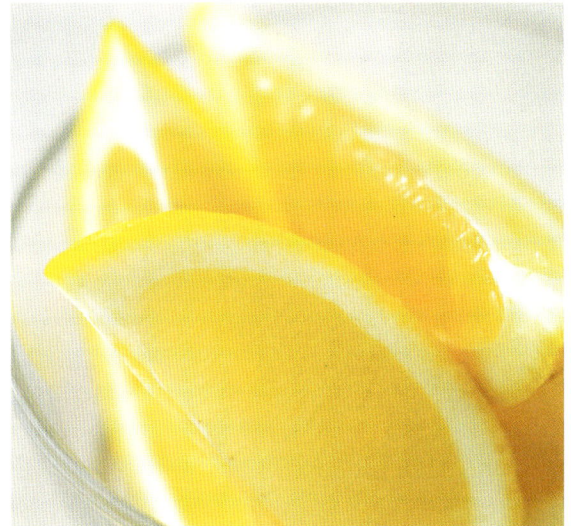

roast chicken and sweet potato with lemon

This fantastic dish can be prepared in advance, is very simple to make and is always greeted with enthusiasm.

2 chickens, each cut into 8 pieces
2 tablespoons light olive oil
2 large kumara (orange sweet potatoes), cut into 3cm cubes
1 teaspoon cumin seeds
1 tablespoon fresh rosemary leaves
2 lemons, thinly sliced

Preheat oven to 200°C. Heat 1 tablespoon of the oil in a large frying pan until really hot. Brown the chicken well, cooking a few pieces at a time. (You can brown the chicken well in advance and keep in the fridge until ready to roast.)

Toss the kumara with the rest of the oil and the cumin seeds and divide between 2 ovenproof dishes. Place the thighs, drumsticks and wings on top of the kumara cubes. Sprinkle with rosemary and place the slices of lemon in with the chicken. Cook in the oven for 30 minutes, then add the pieces of breast and cook for another 30 minutes. Serve with a big salad. Serves 8.

grilled chicken with eggplant salad

4 chicken breast fillets
2 teaspoons extra-virgin olive oil to rub over chicken
3 teaspoons Moroccan spice mixture
2 medium eggplants, thinly sliced
1/4 cup tahini
1/4 cup low-fat yoghurt
2 tablespoons lemon juice
2 teaspoons ground cumin
1 clove garlic, crushed
2 tablespoons extra-virgin olive oil
1 teaspoon sweet paprika
1/3 cup pine nuts, lightly toasted
1/2 cup fresh coriander leaves

Preheat a chargrill pan or barbecue. Rub the chicken fillets with the olive oil and pat with the Moroccan spice mixture. Cook for 4–5 minutes on each side or until cooked. Keep warm until ready to serve.

Place the slices of eggplant in a steamer and steam for 5–7 minutes or until tender. While the eggplant is cooking, combine the tahini, yoghurt, lemon juice, cumin, garlic and olive oil.

Slice the chicken and place with the eggplant on a serving platter. Drizzle over the tahini yoghurt mixture and scatter with the toasted pine nuts and coriander. Serves 4–6.

eggplant, couscous and fetta balls

These delicious eggplant and fetta balls can be made ahead of time and kept in the fridge until you're ready to cook them. They are a bit fiddly to make, but well worth the effort.

balls
1 medium eggplant
1 lemon, juiced
1 onion, finely chopped
100g fetta, crumbled
1 tablespoon freshly grated parmesan
1/2 cup couscous, cooked
1 cup of coarse wholemeal breadcrumbs
1 egg
sea salt and black pepper
light olive or coconut oil for frying

crumb mixture
1/2 cup plain flour
1 egg
1 tablespoon milk (cow, oat or coconut)
1 cup wholemeal breadcrumbs
1 tablespoon parsley, finely chopped
1 tablespoon sesame seeds

Cover pricked eggplant in cold salted water in a saucepan and simmer until eggplant begins to soften (about 20 minutes). Remove from water and peel skin off. Squeeze excess liquid from the flesh and roughly chop. Add lemon juice, onion, fetta, parmesan, couscous, breadcrumbs, egg and salt and pepper. Combine well. Mixture should be wet but easily formed into balls. Divide into 12 round balls and refrigerate for an hour.

To crumb the balls, whisk the egg with milk. Mix breadcrumbs with parsley and sesame seeds. Roll each eggplant ball in the flour, then the egg mixture, then the crumb mixture. Refrigerate until needed.

To cook, heat enough oil to cover the eggplant balls. Fry for a couple of minutes over a medium heat until balls are golden brown. Drain off excess oil on paper towels and serve hot with a crispy green salad. Serves 3–4.

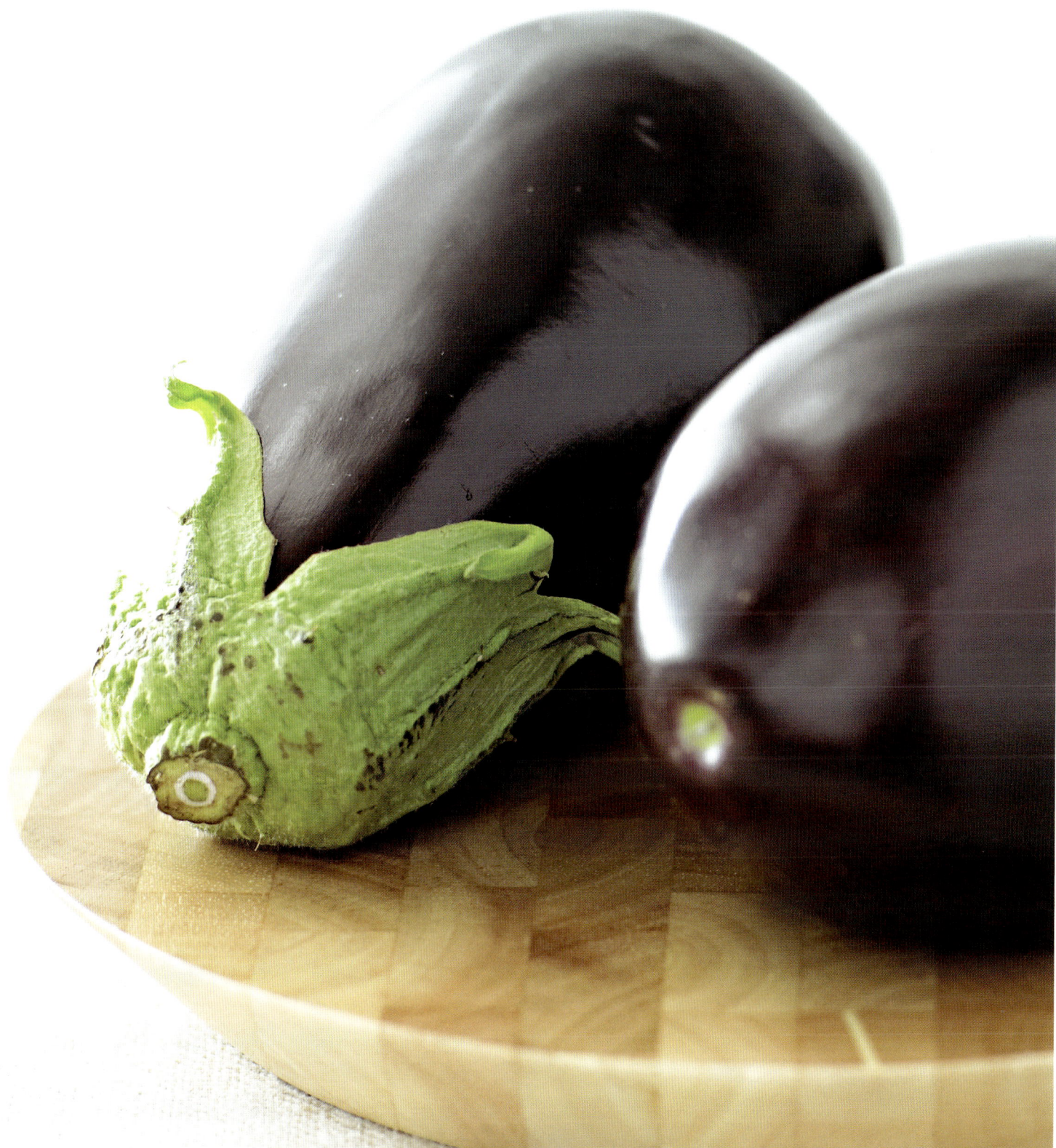

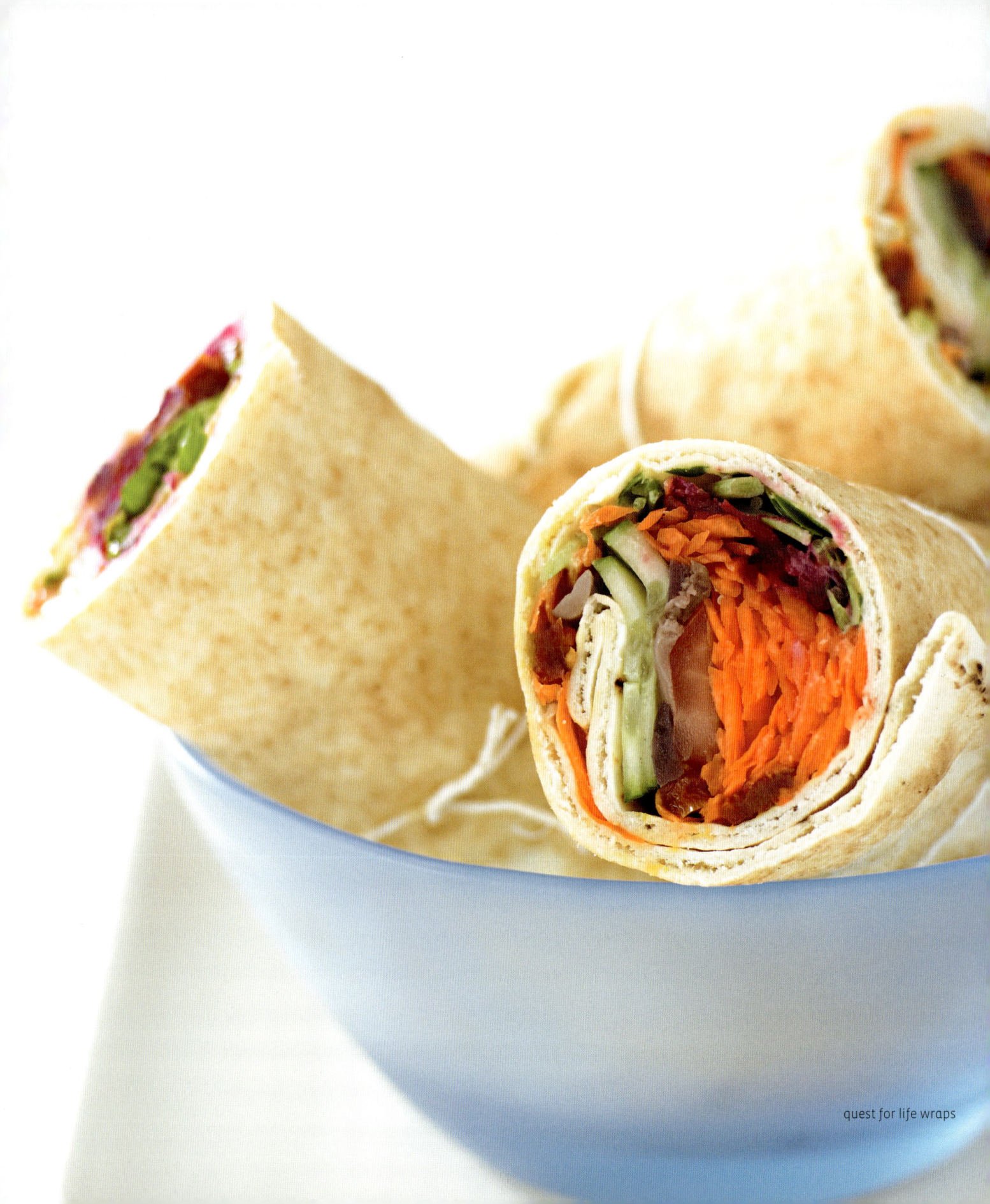

quest for life wraps

Homemade hommus is simple to make and packed with goodness. If you like your hommus light and very smooth, add a little extra yoghurt or the cooking water from the chickpeas. You can also vary the amount of lemon juice. The salad vegetables can be whatever takes your fancy or is in the fridge! If you are pressed for time, use store-bought hommus (without preservatives).

hommus
1 cup chickpeas, soaked overnight, rinsed and simmered
   until soft (or canned)
1/2 cup plain yoghurt
1/4 cup lemon juice
2 tablespoons tahini
1 tablespoon ground cumin
1 clove garlic, crushed

wraps
4 Lebanese breads or pitas
carrot, grated
beetroot, grated
cucumber, sliced
red or green capsicum, thinly sliced
lettuce or salad leaves or rocket, shredded
bean sprouts
tomato, sliced
olives, pitted and sliced
sun-dried tomatoes, sliced

To make the hommus, place all the ingredients in a food processor and blend until smooth.

To make the wraps, spread the flat breads liberally with hommus, then top with salad ingredients of your choice. Roll up tightly and wrap in foil or cling wrap to hold firm. Serves 4.

hoisin chicken with spinach rice

The longer you marinate the chicken before cooking the greater the flavour.

4 chicken breast fillets, sliced in half horizontally
1 tablespoon tamari or soy sauce
1 tablespoon honey
1/4 cup hoisin sauce
2 teaspoons sesame oil
3 cups steamed brown or basmati rice
2 bunches English spinach, steamed and finely chopped
pinch ground nutmeg
sliced green onions (shallots) to serve

Place the sliced chicken in a shallow dish. Combine the tamari, honey and hoisin sauce and pour over the chicken. Cover and marinate for 30 minutes.

Heat a large frying pan and add the sesame oil. Cook the chicken for 3–4 minutes on each side or until cooked.

Combine the rice, chopped spinach and nutmeg and spoon onto 4 plates. Top with the chicken and sliced green onions. Serves 4.

Organic fruit and vegetables have increased levels of vitamins, minerals, anti-oxidants and other essential nutrients. Always use ripe and seasonal fruit to maximise the flavour.

lime chicken with mint raita

800g chicken, cut into strips
1/2 cup fresh lime juice
3 cloves garlic, crushed
1 teaspoon ground fennel seeds
1 tablespoon extra-virgin olive oil
2 cups plain yoghurt
1 bunch mint leaves

Place the chicken in a bowl and combine with the lime juice, garlic and fennel seeds. Marinate for 20 minutes then thread onto wooden skewers. Brush with oil and grill or barbecue until golden and cooked.

For the mint raita, remove the mint leaves from the stalks and place in a food processor or blender. Add the yoghurt and a pinch of sea salt. Blend until smooth. Serve with the chicken. Serves 8.

chicken kebabs with pear salsa

800g chicken breast fillets
3 teaspoons sesame oil
2 teaspoons ground coriander
2 teaspoons ground cumin

pear salsa
2 just ripe pears, finely diced
1/2 Spanish (red) onion, finely chopped
1 stick celery, finely diced

dressing
1 tablespoon chopped chives
2 tablespoons lemon juice
2 teaspoons Dijon mustard
1/2 avocado, peeled and stone removed
3/4 cup water

100g soft mixed lettuce leaves to serve

Cut the chicken into 3cm pieces and toss in the oil, coriander and cumin. Thread onto 8 skewers and heat a barbecue or grill. Cook the kebabs over medium heat, turning occasionally for 6–8 minutes or until cooked. Loosely cover and keep warm while you prepare the salsa.

For the salsa, combine the pears, red onion and celery. For the dressing, place the chives, lemon juice, mustard, avocado and water in a food processor and blend until smooth. Place the lettuce on a serving platter with the kebabs on top. Drizzle with the dressing and serve with the pear salsa. Serves 4.

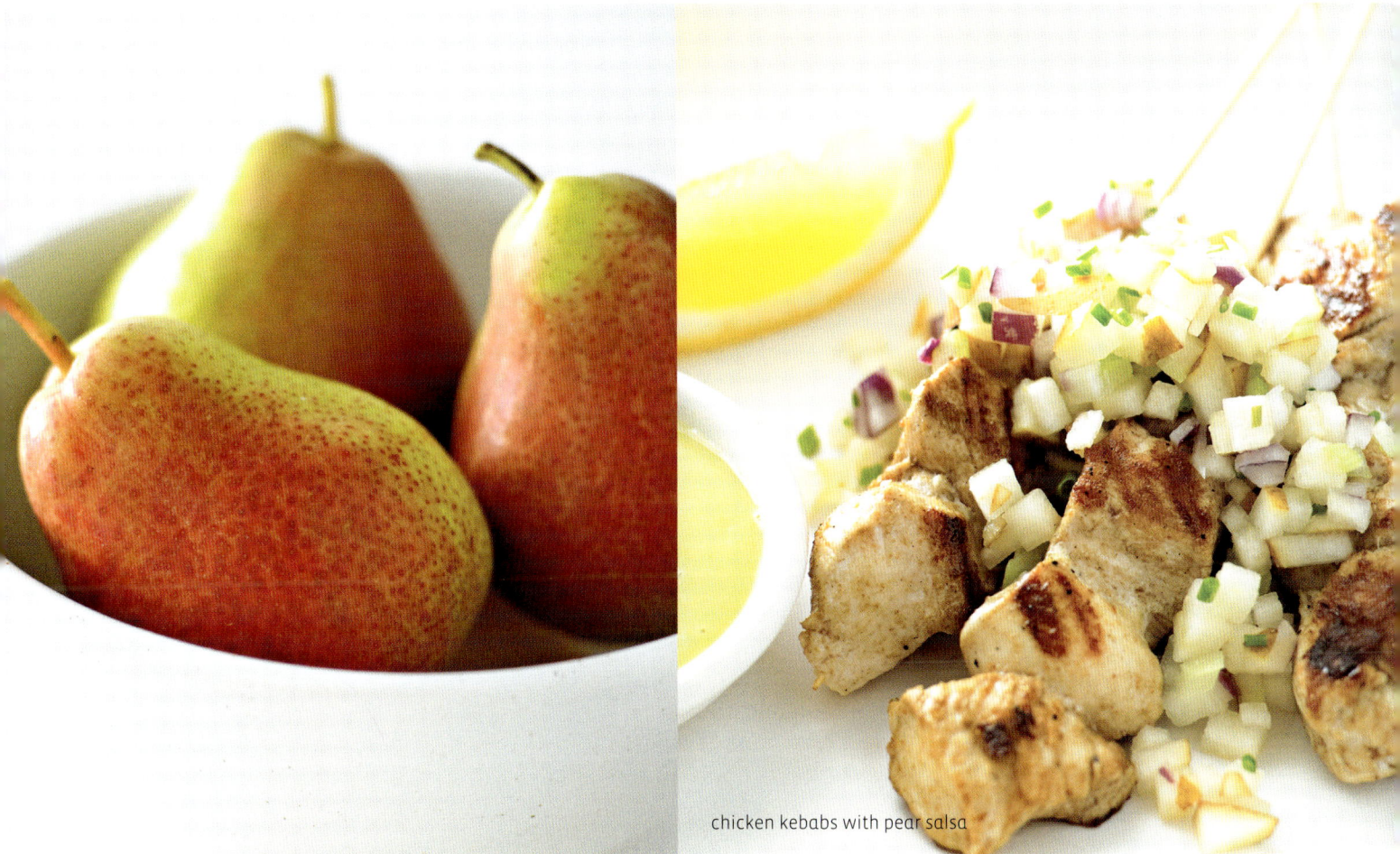

chicken kebabs with pear salsa

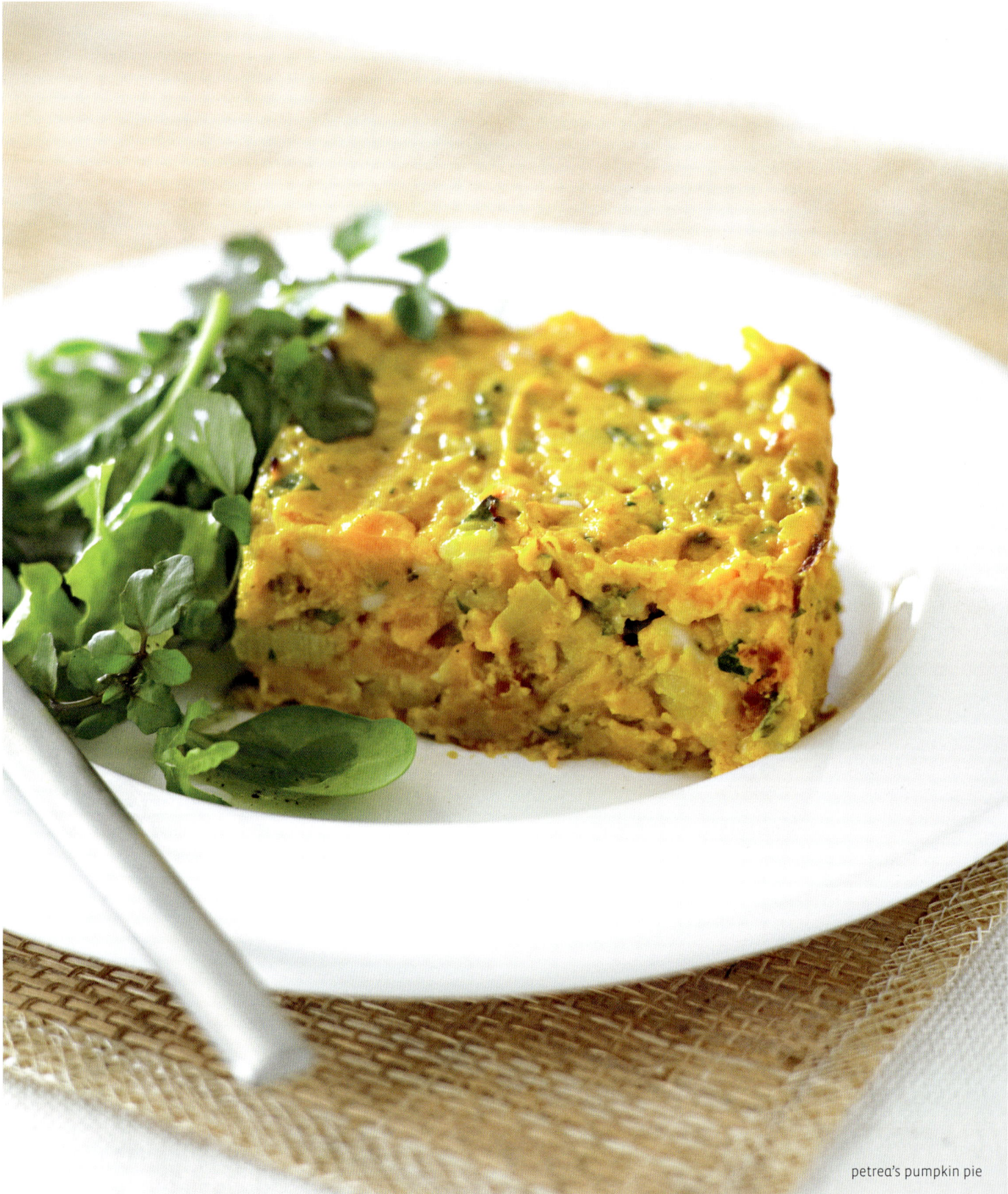

petrea's pumpkin pie

middle eastern wraps

This is a great favourite with families as everyone seems able to find something they like. Eating with hands also makes everyone feel relaxed. I'm only giving you the recipe for the tabouli as all the other ingredients you can buy or prepare very simply and homemade tabouli is so much better than any you can buy.

2 cups kalamata olives, for nibbling
whole almonds and roast pistachios, for nibbling
16 Lebanese breads
1–2 cups hommus (see page 97)
1–2 cups babaganoush (eggplant dip)
12 falafels (chickpea patties)
8 chicken breast fillets or 12 thighs, sprinkled with
    Moroccan spice mixture, barbecued or grilled, then sliced
400g fetta cheese, cut into cubes

tabouli
¼ cup burghul (cracked wheat)
2 bunches flat-leaf parsley, stalks removed and leaves
    finely chopped
1 bunch mint, stalks removed and leaves chopped
8 green onions (shallots), finely chopped
4 tomatoes, diced
1 cucumber, finely diced
1 lemon, juiced
¼ cup extra-virgin olive oil
1 teaspoon ground black pepper
½ teaspoon mixed spice (Lebanese if possible)

To make the tabouli, rinse the burghul in a sieve, drain and place in a large mixing bowl. Add the chopped parsley, mint, green onions, tomatoes and cucumber and combine. Drizzle with the lemon juice and oil and stir through the spices. Pile into 2 bowls and put one at each end of the table.

Wrap the Lebanese breads in foil and warm in a 180°C oven for 15 minutes. (If the bread is very fresh you don't need to warm.)

Place all the other foods in bowls and on platters. Serves 8.

petrea's pumpkin pie

My children, Kate and Simon, were raised as vegetarians and this recipe was their all-time favourite. Even now we rarely have a family gathering where this dish doesn't feature. It is also a great favourite at the Quest for Life Centre. Pumpkin is a great source of potassium and folate and this recipe is naturally sweet and filling. Other vegetables can be added to the basic recipe for variety.

1kg pumpkin, cooked and mashed
1 tablespoon sesame or extra-virgin olive oil
1 tablespoon unsalted butter
2 leeks, sliced or two large onions, diced
3 cloves garlic, diced
8 eggs, lightly beaten
500gm low-fat cottage cheese
¼ cup honey (optional)
2 teaspoons nutmeg
2 tablespoons dried mixed herbs
1 cup finely chopped fresh mixed herbs
sea salt and black pepper

Preheat the oven to 220°C. Heat the oil in a frying pan and add the leek or onions and garlic. (A cup of sliced zucchinis, diced broccoli or cauliflower heads or other vegetables can also be added.) Sauté until soft.

Combine the mashed pumpkin with the remaining ingredients. Pour into an ovenproof dish and bake for 30 minutes covered with foil, then 30 minutes uncovered or until firm and golden. Serves 6–8.

vegetable kebabs with plum sauce

The delicious plum sauce used here is available from many supermarkets and Asian grocery stores.

8 small yellow squash, halved
8 cherry tomatoes
8 small mushrooms
1 Spanish (red) onion, cut into wedges
200g firm tempeh, cut into 3cm cubes
1 tablespoon extra-virgin olive oil
1/3 cup plum sauce, warmed
1 tablespoon chopped fresh dill
3 cups cooked basmati rice

Thread the vegetables and tempeh onto 8 wooden or metal skewers and brush with oil. Heat a large frying pan and cook the kebabs over medium heat until the vegetables are tender. Pour over the plum sauce.

Scatter over the chopped dill and serve with basmati rice. Serves 4.

asian noodle salad

If you don't want to use fish sauce then substitute with tamari or soy sauce. It might seem like a fair amount of chopping and slicing of vegetables but it's definitely worth the effort.

salad
300g rice noodles
1/2 red cabbage, shredded
1/4 Chinese cabbage, shredded
100g snow pea sprouts, trimmed
150g snow peas, trimmed and blanched
150g green beans, trimmed and blanched
1/2 red capsicum, seeded and finely sliced
1/2 yellow capsicum, seeded and finely sliced
1/2 bunch coriander, chopped

dressing
1/3 cup fish sauce
2 tablespoons mirin
1/3 cup fresh lime juice
1 tablespoon honey or palm sugar

Cook the rice noodles for 2 minutes in boiling water or until tender. Drain, rinse and cut into bite-size lengths with scissors. Combine with all the chopped vegetables and gently toss.

Whisk together the fish sauce, mirin, lime juice and honey or palm sugar. Drizzle over the salad and serve. Serves 4–6.

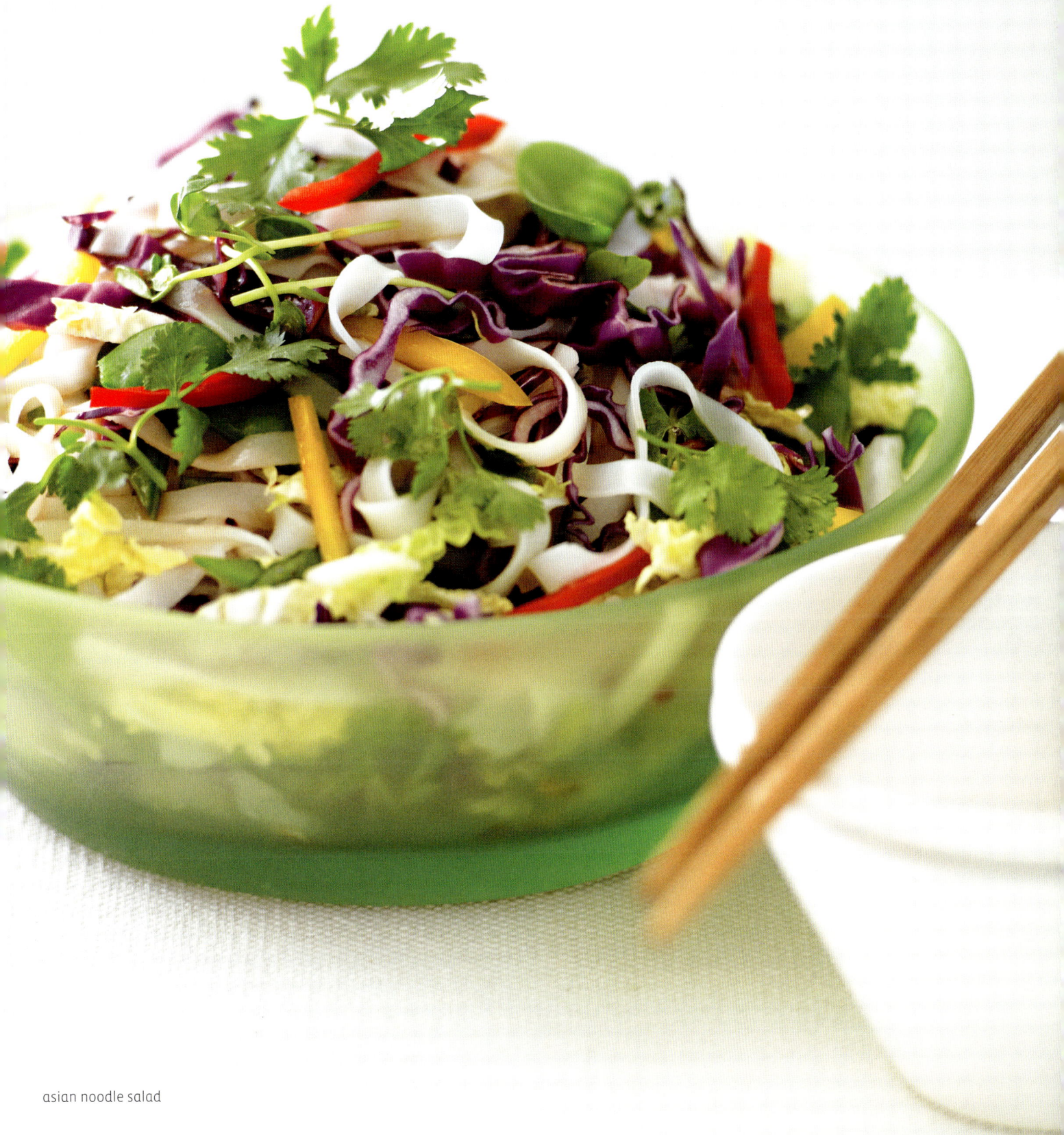

asian noodle salad

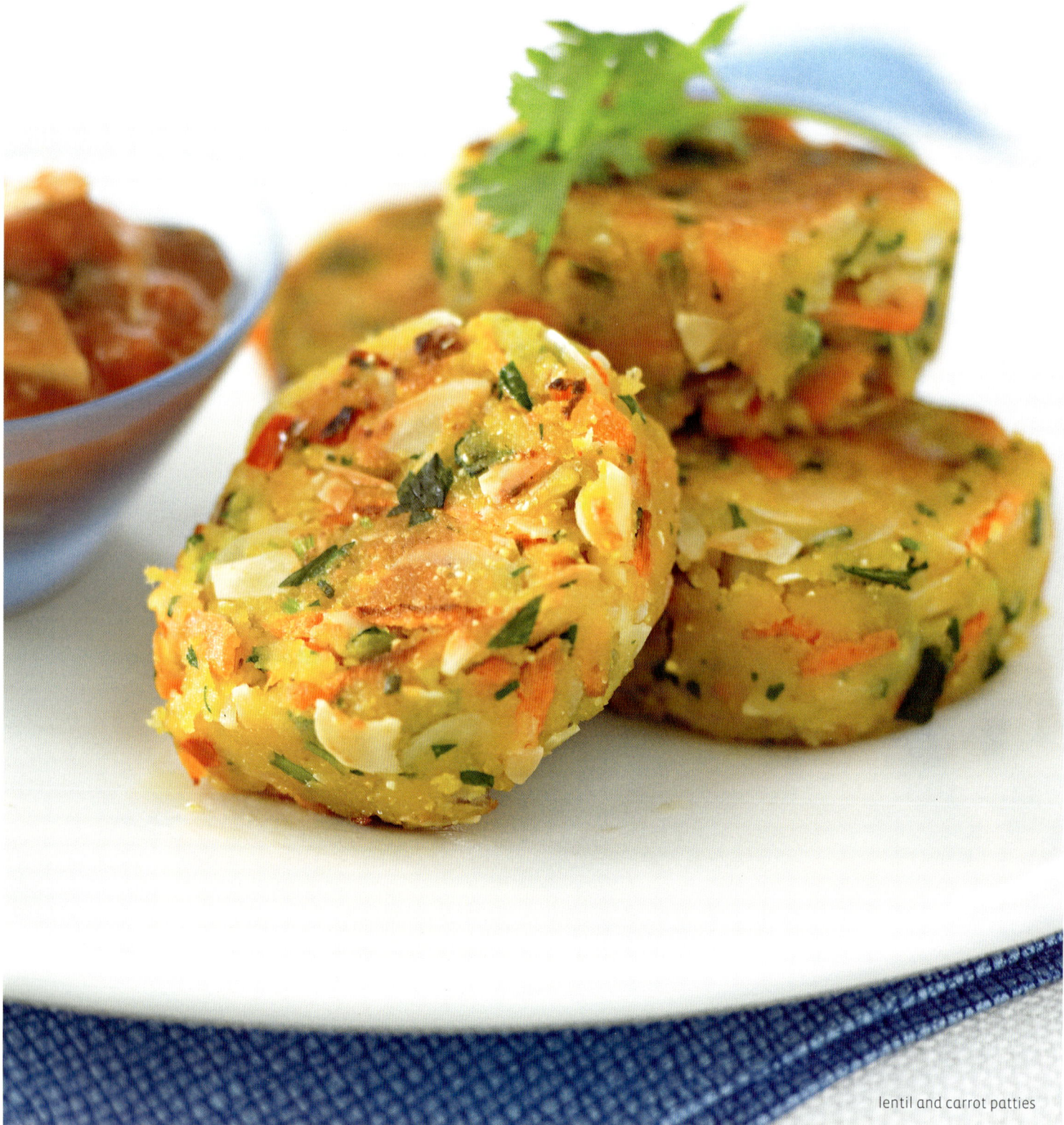

lentil and carrot patties

lentil and carrot patties

Those who are wheat intolerant can omit the breadcrumbs and use polenta instead. Very good served with green tahini (page 113) or sweet chilli sauce.

500g red lentils, washed and drained
1 Spanish (red) onion, finely chopped
500g grated carrot
100g flaked almonds
100g fresh breadcrumbs or ½ cup polenta
1 cup chopped fresh herbs (parsley, oregano, mint, basil, dill etc.)
2 eggs, lightly beaten
1 red chilli, seeded and chopped
sea salt and black pepper
sesame oil or extra-virgin olive oil
lemon wedges for serving

Place the lentils in a saucepan and cover with cold water. Bring to the boil and simmer for 15 minutes or until soft. Drain well and place in a large bowl. Combine with the onion, carrot, almonds, breadcrumbs or polenta, herbs, eggs, chilli and salt and pepper. Place in the fridge for 1 hour to firm up.

Using a spoon and one hand, form the mixture into patties. Heat a large frying pan and add a little sesame oil. Fry the patties in batches until golden and cooked. Serve with lemon wedges and salsa (recipe follows). Serves 4.

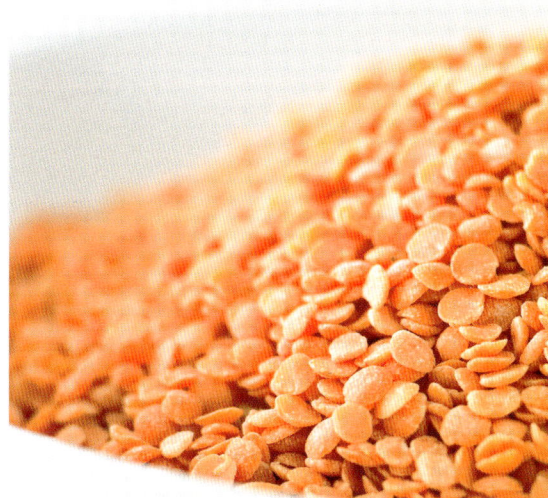

doug's vegetable salsa

This salsa is fabulous with the red lentil and carrot patties, but is very versatile. Try it with hot tempeh, grilled chicken or fish or spooned over chickpeas or kidney or other beans.

3 teaspoons extra-virgin olive oil
1 leek, chopped
1 clove garlic, crushed
100g mushrooms, chopped
400g can crushed tomatoes
1 tablespoon tomato paste
1 tablespoon honey
2 tablespoons chopped basil
sea salt and black pepper

Heat a frying pan and add the olive oil. Add the leek and cook over medium heat until soft. Stir through the garlic and mushrooms and cook until the mushrooms are soft.

Add the tomatoes and tomato paste, honey and basil and bring to the boil. Reduce the heat and simmer for 10 minutes. Season with sea salt and black pepper. Cool and then place in the fridge. Can be served hot or cold. Makes 1 cup.

spinach and ricotta cannelloni

There's nothing more tempting at the market than piles of green spinach. Just looking at it convinces you of its health benefits. The secret of this deliciously simple recipe is to use fresh lasagne sheets which you'll find in the chilled section of the supermarket.

tomato sauce
1 tablespoon extra-virgin olive oil
1 onion, finely chopped
1 clove garlic, finely chopped
2 x 400g cans crushed tomatoes
2 tablespoons tomato paste
sea salt and black pepper

cannelloni
3 bunches English spinach, washed, trimmed, roughly
   chopped, steamed and squeezed dry
500g fresh ricotta
2 eggs, lightly beaten
1/2 teaspoon ground nutmeg
1/4 teaspoon ground mace
8 green onions (shallots), thinly sliced
6 fresh lasagne sheets, halved
1/2 cup freshly grated parmesan

Preheat the oven to 200°C and lightly oil 2 medium rectangular baking dishes.

To make the tomato sauce, heat the oil in a saucepan and add the onion. Gently cook for 5 minutes or until soft and golden. Add the garlic and stir. Add the tomatoes and tomato paste and bring to the boil. Reduce the heat, cover and simmer for 10 minutes. Season with salt and pepper.

Combine the cooked spinach, ricotta, eggs, nutmeg, mace and green onions in a large bowl. Place one twelfth of the mixture on each sheet of lasagne, form into a log the length of the sheet and roll up. Repeat with the remaining mixture until you have 12 cannelloni.

Place a couple of spoons of tomato sauce in each baking dish. Place 6 cannelloni in each dish and top with the remaining tomato mixture, thoroughly covering the pasta. Sprinkle with the cheese and tightly cover with foil. Bake in the oven for 40 minutes or until cooked. Serves 4–6.

pumpkin and mushroom risotto

Hearty and comforting, risotto is perfect for an easy winter's meal. The slow stirring of the rice and stock is very soothing and the sweet and earthy favour of the pumpkin and mushrooms is simply delicious.

15g dried porcini mushrooms
250g button mushrooms, quartered
2 tablespoons extra-virgin olive oil
1 onion, finely chopped
250g pumpkin, cut into 1.5cm cubes
about 7 cups hot vegetable stock
2 cups arborio rice
75g freshly grated Parmesan

Soak the porcini in 1 cup of near boiling water for 15 minutes. Drain, reserving the soaking liquid to combine with the stock, and finely chop the porcini. Panfry the quartered fresh mushrooms with a drop of oil and reserve.

Heat the olive oil in a large, heavy-based saucepan. Add the onion and cook for 2–3 minutes. Add the pumpkin and cook for 5 minutes or until nearly tender. Add the rice and porcini to the saucepan and cook for 1 minute while stirring.

Combine the stock and the porcini soaking liquid in another saucepan and simmer. Stir a ladle of hot stock into the rice mixture and stir until the liquid is absorbed. Continue adding the stock and stirring, one ladleful at a time, until the rice is creamy and cooked. Add more stock if necessary. Stir through the cooked button mushrooms and grated parmesan and serve in warm bowls. Serves 4.

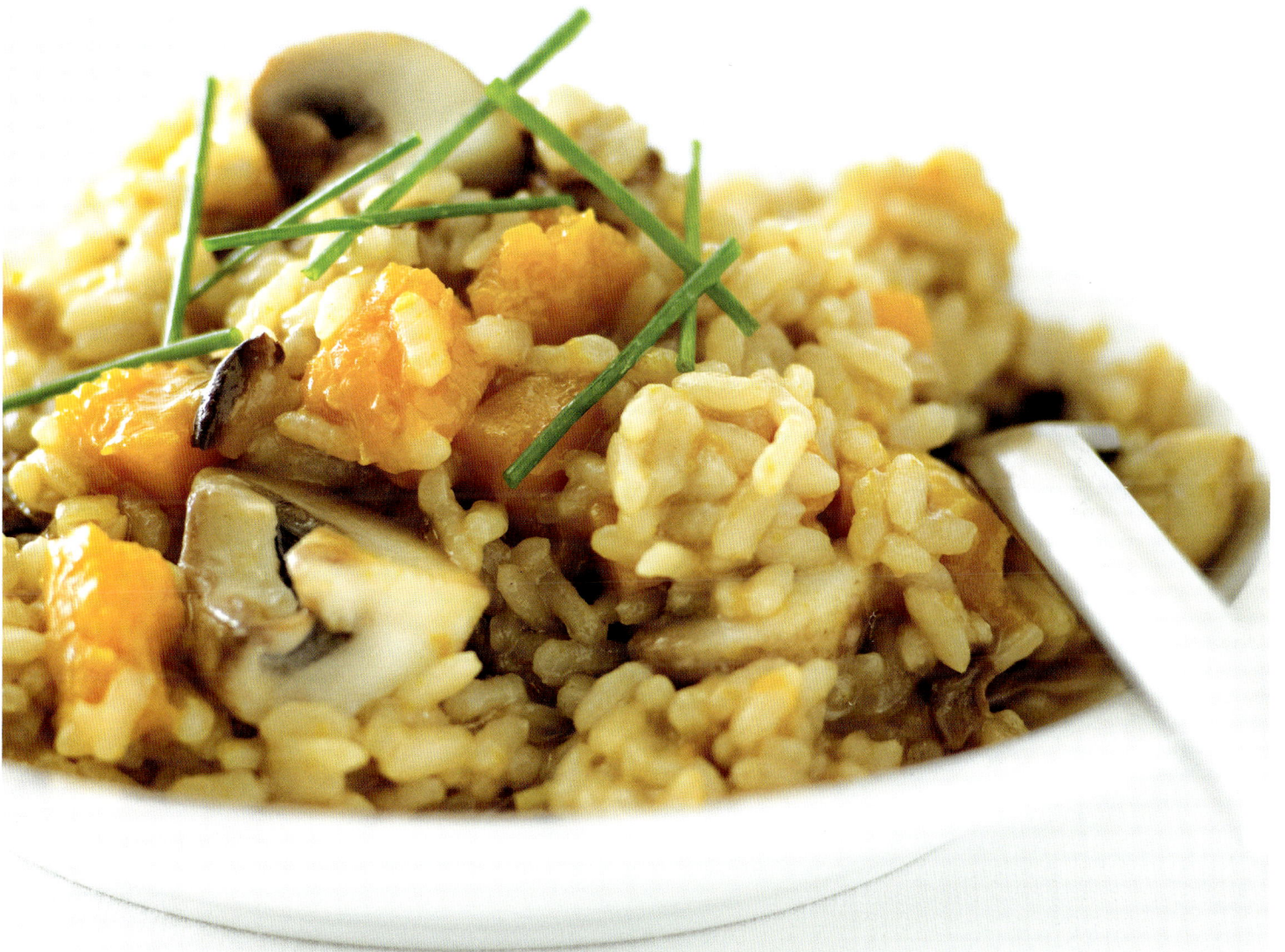

pumpkin and mushroom risotto

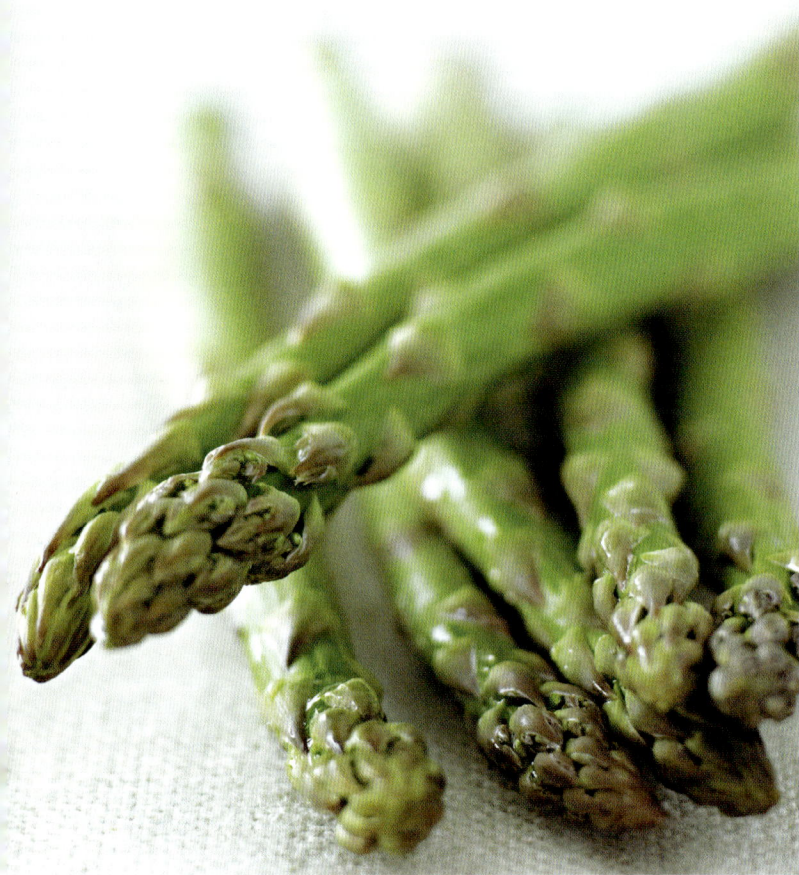

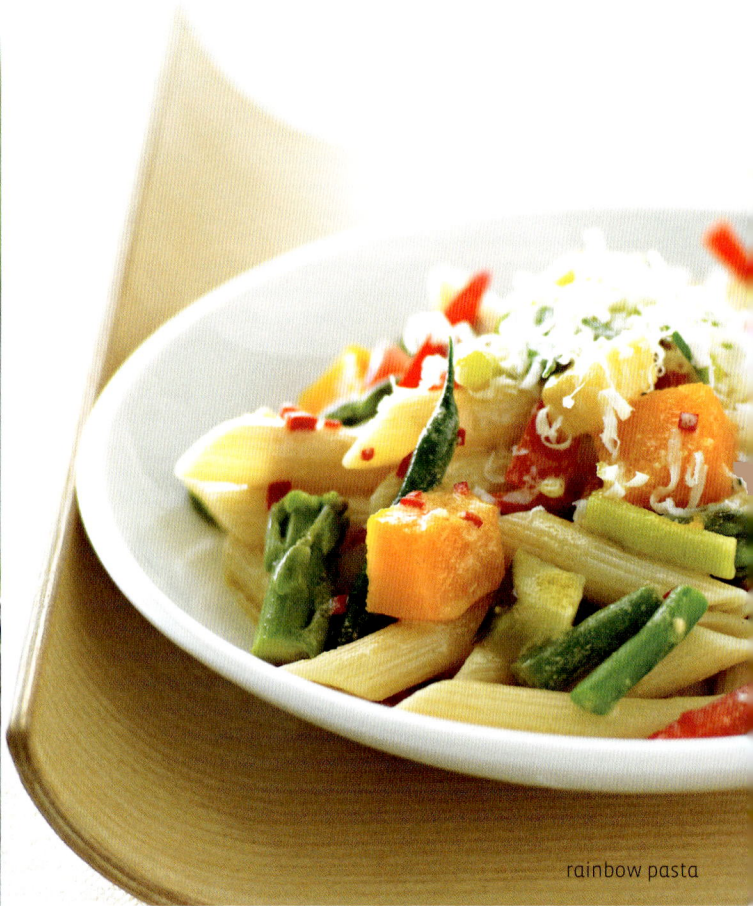

rainbow pasta

avocado and basil pesto pasta with roast tomatoes

When basil is in season make the most of the big, fragrant bunches of this delicious herb. This pesto sauce is just as good as the traditional one but without the copious quantities of oil and cheese.

250g cherry or truss tomatoes
2 teaspoons extra-virgin olive oil
$1/4$ cup pine nuts
2 bunches fresh basil leaves
$1/3$ cup lemon juice
1 clove garlic, crushed
1 large ripe avocado, peeled and seed removed
sea salt and black pepper
$1/2$ cup water
400g wholemeal, regular or wheat-free pasta

Heat the oven to 200°C. Toss the tomatoes in olive oil and place on a baking tray. Bake for 15 minutes or until soft.

Place the pine nuts, basil, lemon juice and garlic in a food processor. Blend until combined. Add the avocado, water, salt and black pepper and continue to blend until smooth.

Cook the pasta in boiling water until tender. Stir through the pesto sauce and top with the roasted tomatoes. Serves 4.

There's nothing like al dente pasta with fresh seasonal vegetables for a quick, satisfying, tasty meal.

rainbow pasta

500g dried penne
1 bunch asparagus, trimmed and cut into 4cm lengths
150g green and yellow beans, cut into bite-size lengths
1 cup diced eggplant
1 red capsicum, seeded and finely sliced
4 tomatoes, seeded and diced
$1/4$ cup extra-virgin olive oil
  or $1/4$ –$1/2$ cup hot vegetable stock
$1/4$ cup lemon juice
2 teaspoons Dijon mustard
1 teaspoon chopped red chilli (optional)
sea salt and black pepper
$1/3$ cup freshly grated parmesan

Cook the pasta in boiling water until just tender. While the pasta is cooking, steam the asparagus, beans and eggplant then place in a large warm bowl. Toss together with the red capsicum and diced tomato and cooked pasta.

Whisk together the olive oil, lemon juice, mustard and chilli (if using). Gently toss through the pasta and vegetable mixture and season with sea salt and black pepper. Scatter with grated parmesan and serve. Serves 4.

spinach, mushroom and corn casserole

1 tablespoon extra-virgin olive oil
1 onion, finely chopped
2 cloves garlic, chopped
200g mushrooms, chopped
1 bunch silver beet, stalks removed, washed and shredded
kernels from 2 corn cobs
$\frac{1}{4}$ teaspoon ground nutmeg
500g fresh ricotta, crumbled
1 egg, lightly beaten
6 sheets filo pastry
sea salt and black pepper
2 teaspoons extra-virgin olive oil, extra

Heat oven to 200°C. Brush a 20cmx20cm baking dish with olive oil. Heat 1 tablespoon of oil in a frying pan and add the onion. Cook over medium heat until soft and golden. Stir through the garlic and mushrooms. Cook until the mushrooms soften.

Blanch the silver beet and corn kernels in boiling water, then transfer to icy water to rapidly cool. Drain excess water. Combine with the onion, garlic and mushroom mixture. Stir through the nutmeg, ricotta and egg. Season the mixture with sea salt and black pepper.

Cover the filo pastry sheets with a damp tea towel. Brush 1 sheet with olive oil, top with another and repeat using remaining sheets and oil. Fold the pile in half and place on top of the vegetable mixture. Tuck any excess filo down the sides of the dish. Cook for 40 minutes or until cooked and golden. Serves 4.

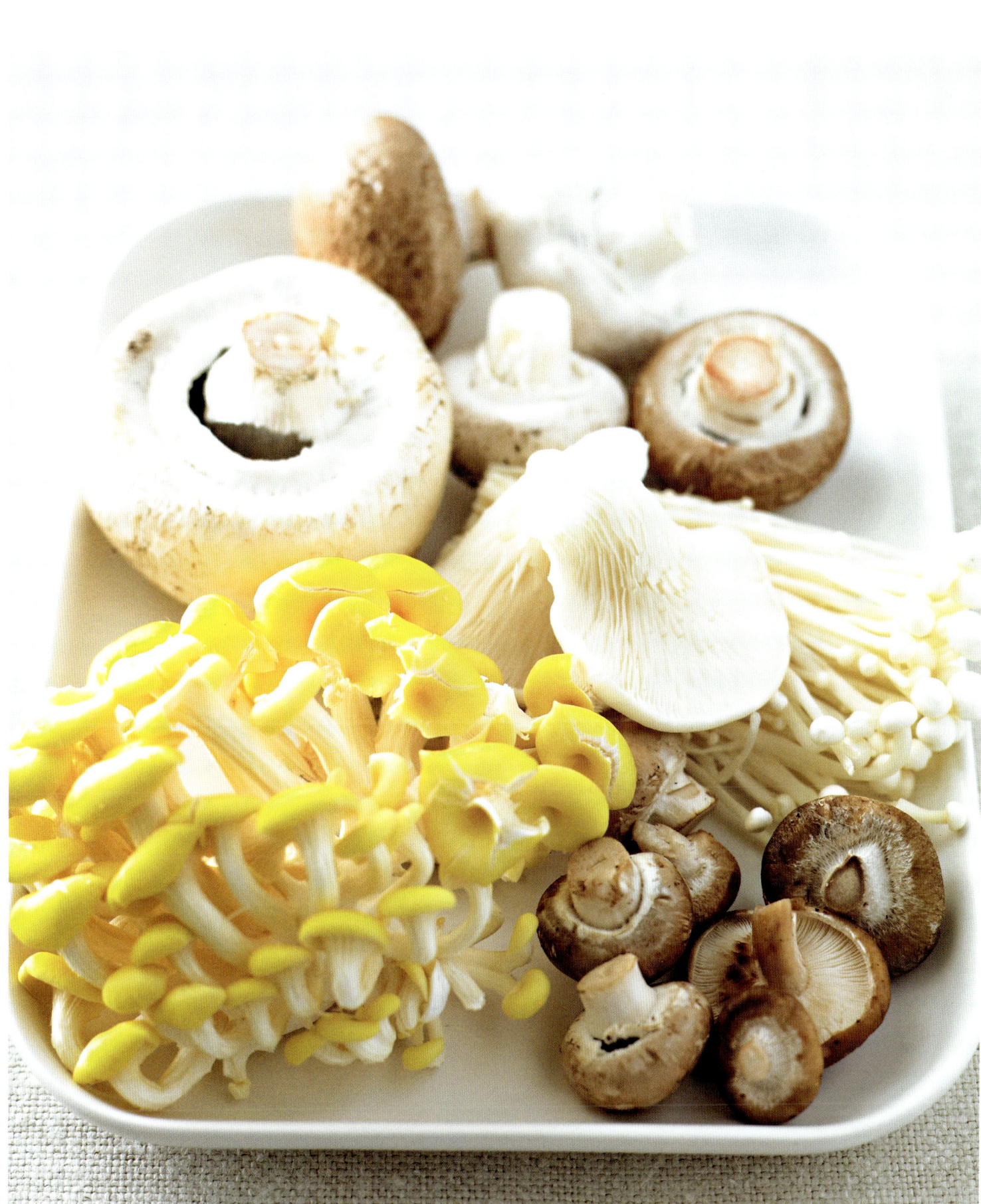

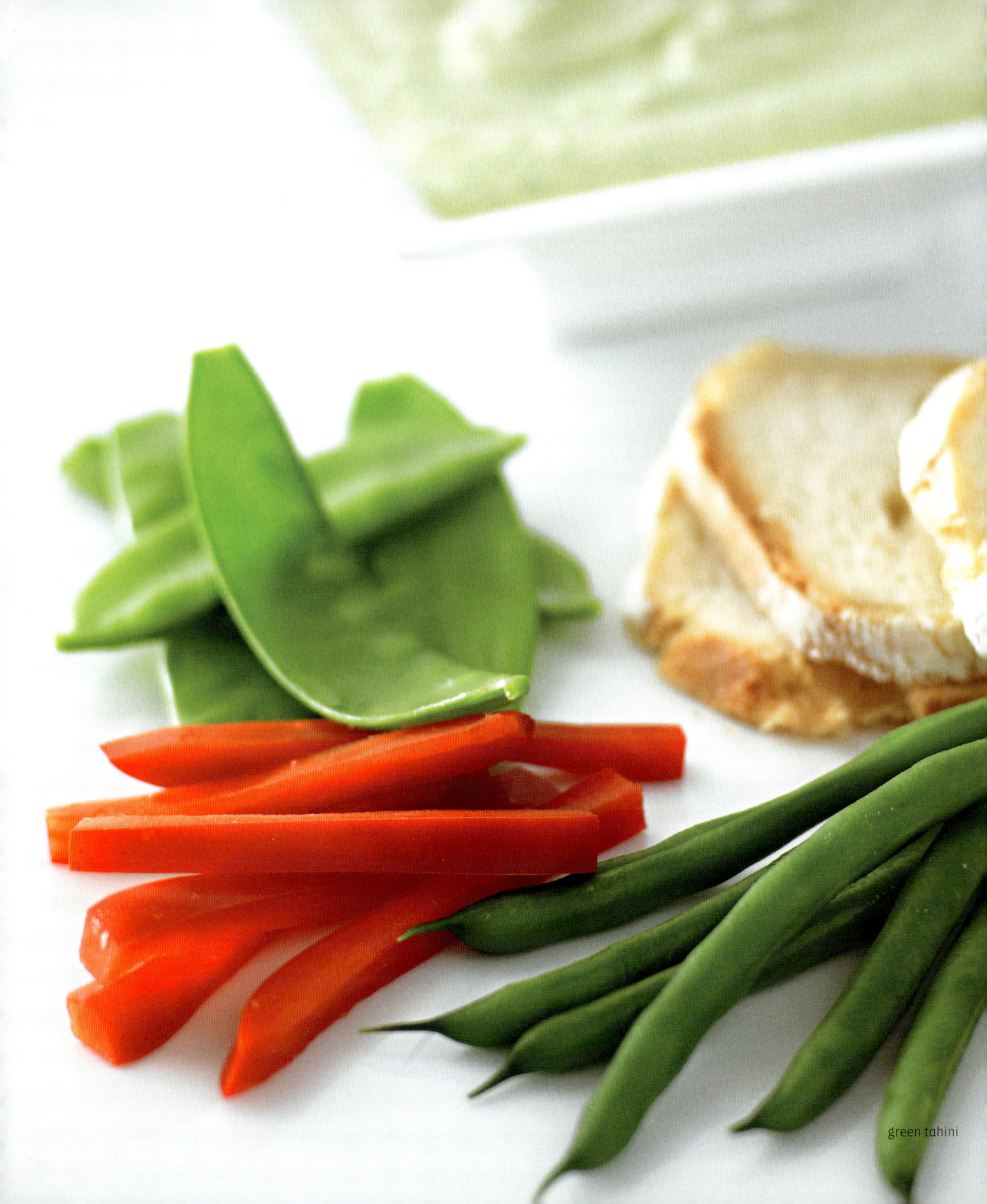

green tahini

green tahini

This colourful and nutritious dip is a wonderful accompaniment to many meals and great with toasted pita bread, raw vegetables or used in wraps.

1/2 cup tahini
juice of 2 lemons
1/4 cup water
1 clove garlic, crushed
1/2 cup roughly chopped coriander
1/4 cup roughly chopped parsley
sea salt and black pepper

Place all the ingredients (except salt and pepper) into a food processor and blend until smooth. Season with sea salt and black pepper and spoon into an airtight container. Store in the fridge for up to a week. Makes 1 cup.

chickpea, pumpkin and tahini casserole

Tahini is a delicious paste made from sesame seeds and it is frequently used in Middle Eastern cookery. Use leftover tahini to make tasty green tahini (preceding recipe).

500g pumpkin, diced into 2cm chunks
2 tablespoons extra-virgin olive oil
2 teaspoons ground cumin
1 onion, finely chopped
2 cloves garlic, crushed
500g cooked chickpeas
1/2 cup tahini
1/2 cup water
1/4 cup lemon juice
1 cup chopped flat-leaf parsley

Preheat the oven to 200°C. Line a baking tray with baking paper. Toss the pumpkin with 1 tablespoon of oil and sprinkle with the cumin. Bake in the oven for 40 minutes or until cooked.

While the pumpkin is cooking, heat the remaining oil in a frying pan. Add the onion and cook over medium heat until soft and golden. Add the garlic and cook for another minute. Add the chickpeas and heat through.

Combine the tahini, water and lemon juice until smooth. Stir into the chickpea mixture along with the pumpkin and parsley. Continue to cook, stirring until the mixture is hot. Season with sea salt and black pepper. Serve with brown rice and salad. Serves 4.

roast vegetable pizza

Just about any vegetable can be roasted and put on top of a pizza. Even roasted green beans and asparagus are delicious! Green vegetables should be added only for the last 10 minutes of cooking.

2 Spanish (red) onions, cut into wedges
1 zucchini, cut into thick slices
1 red capsicum, seeded and cut into 2cm squares
2 cups cubed kumara or pumpkin
12 button mushrooms, quartered
3 tablespoons extra-virgin olive oil
2 cloves garlic, crushed
1 teaspoon dried chilli flakes
4 Lebanese breads
$1/3$ cup tomato paste
slices of bocconcini or grated mozzarella (optional)
3 teaspoons dried oregano
baby rocket leaves to serve

Heat the oven to 200°C. Toss all the vegetables (except baby rocket leaves and garlic) together with the oil and place on a baking tray lined with baking paper. Cook in the oven for 40 minutes then stir through the garlic and chilli flakes.

Turn the oven up to 220°C. Place the Lebanese breads on baking trays (you may need to cook them in 2 batches). Spread evenly with the tomato paste. Top with the roasted vegetables and bocconcini or mozzarella (if using). Sprinkle over the oregano and cook in the oven until the bases are crisp and the cheese has melted (about 12 minutes). Scatter with baby rocket leaves. Serves 4.

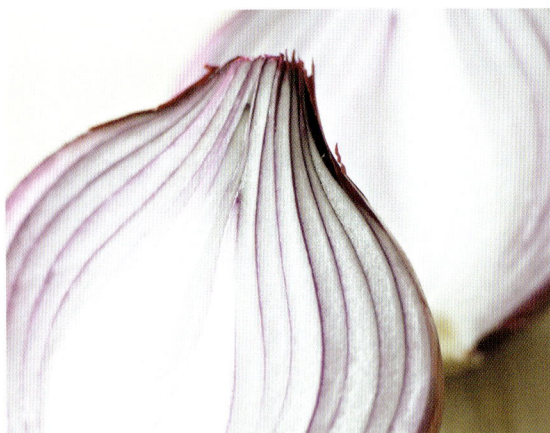

lentil bolognese

If you don't eat pasta or simply want a tasty alternative, then roast diced pumpkin, parsnip, potato or eggplant and spoon over the lentil bolognese.

1 tablespoon extra-virgin olive oil
1 leek, chopped
1 stick celery, finely chopped
1 carrot, finely chopped
1 teaspoon cumin seeds
$1^1/2$ cups red lentils, rinsed and drained
400g can chopped tomatoes
1 cup vegetable stock or water
$1/4$ cup tomato paste
3 teaspoons dried oregano
400g dried spaghetti
sea salt and black pepper
freshly grated parmesan to serve (optional)

Heat the oil in a large frying pan and add the leek, celery and carrot. Cook over medium heat until softened. Add the cumin seeds and red lentils and stir until well combined.

Add the tomatoes, vegetable stock or water, tomato paste and oregano. Bring to the boil, then reduce the heat and simmer covered for 20 minutes. Season with sea salt and black pepper.

While the lentil bolognese is cooking, cook the spaghetti in boiling water until tender. Drain and serve with the bolognese. Scatter with grated parmesan (if using). Serves 4.

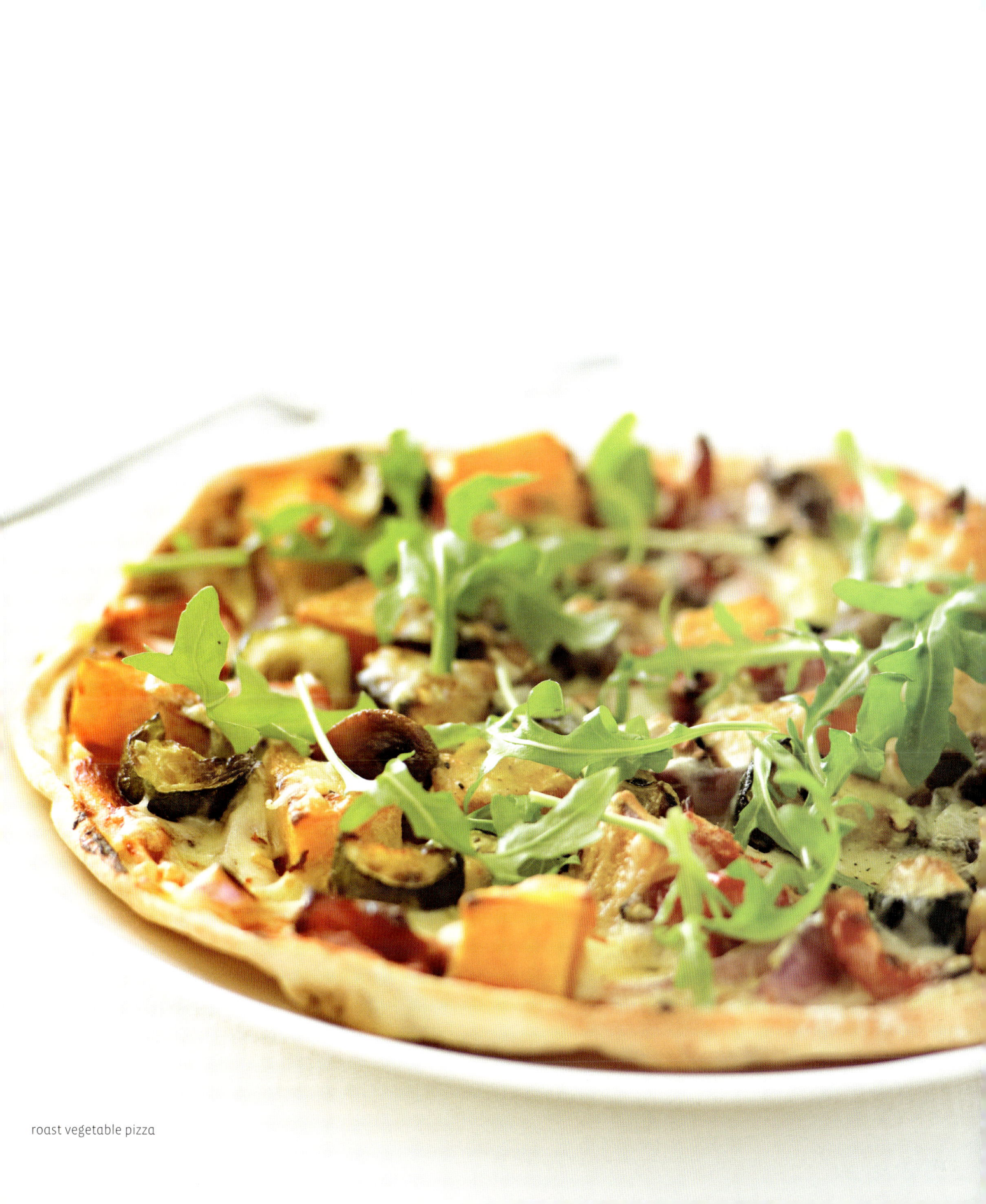

roast vegetable pizza

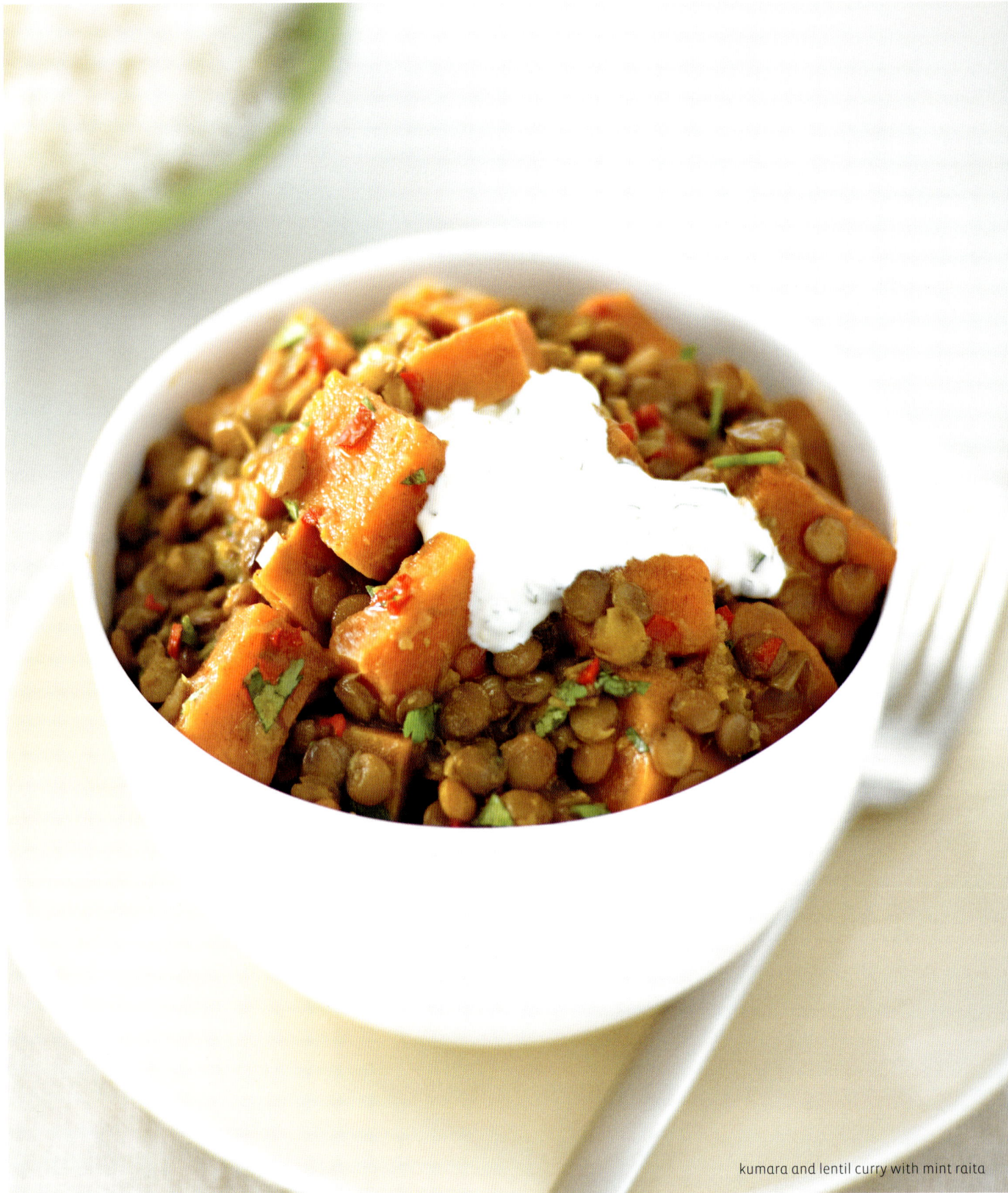

kumara and lentil curry with mint raita

kumara and lentil curry with mint raita

Kumara, the sweet potato with orange-coloured flesh, is high in fibre, vitamin A and other antioxidants. It also tastes great in a curry.

3 tablespoons Indian curry paste
1 cup brown lentils, rinsed and drained
2 bay leaves
500g kumara, peeled and diced
1 tablespoon grated fresh ginger
1 teaspoon chopped red chilli (optional)
2¹/₂ cups vegetable stock
¹/₄ cup chopped coriander
sea salt

raita
¹/₂ cup mint leaves
1 cup plain yoghurt
1 teaspoon grated fresh ginger
1 clove garlic, crushed
¹/₂ cup finely chopped cucumber

Heat a saucepan and add the curry paste. Cook over low heat for 1 minute, while stirring. Add the lentils, bay leaves, sweet potato, ginger, chilli (if using) and vegetable stock. Bring to the boil then reduce the heat and simmer covered for 35–40 minutes or until the lentils and kumara are tender. Add more stock if necessary. Stir through the coriander and season with sea salt.

While the curry is cooking, make the raita. Place the mint leaves, ginger, yoghurt and garlic in a food processor or blender. Blend until smooth then mix through chopped cucumber just before serving. Pour into a bowl and enjoy with the curry. Serves 4.

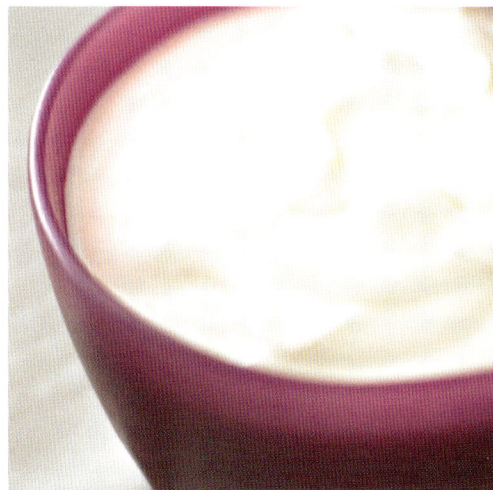

lentil and vegetable curry

1 tablespoon sesame or coconut oil
2 onions, chopped
2 tablespoons finely chopped fresh ginger
¹/₂ cup Indian curry paste (e.g. Rogan Josh)
3¹/₂ cups vegetable stock
400ml can coconut milk
3 cups pumpkin, peeled and cut into 2cm cubes
1¹/₂ cups red lentils, rinsed and drained
4 cups sliced vegetables (snow peas, green beans, potato, zucchinis, carrots etc.)
¹/₂ cup fresh coriander leaves
basmati rice with spinach, pappadums and mango chutney to serve

Heat the oil in a large saucepan then add the onion. Gently cook until soft and golden. Add the ginger and curry paste and cook for another minute.

Add the vegetable stock, coconut milk, pumpkin and lentils. Bring to the boil, then reduce the heat and simmer for 15 minutes. Add the sliced vegetables and cook for another 5 minutes or until tender.

Serve with basmati rice folded together with finely chopped spinach, pappadums and mango chutney. Serves 8.

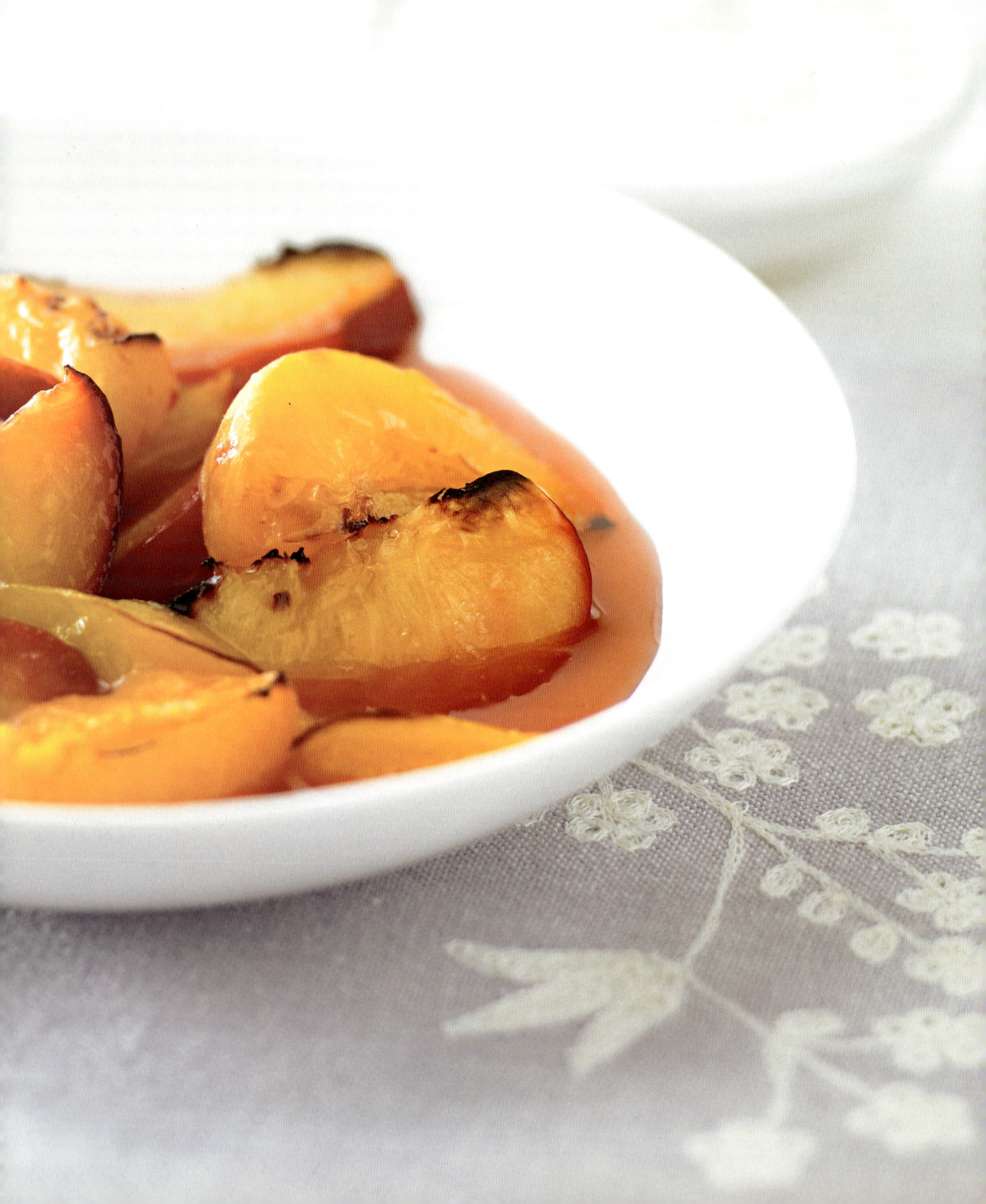

Desserts

desserts

While fresh or dried fruit is great for satisfying a sweet tooth, many people find that they crave a special treat! The following recipes will satisfy any sweet desires as well as being fun to make.

OVER THE PAST hundred years the annual consumption of sugar in Australia has soared. At the beginning of the twentieth century we consumed about half a kilogram of sugar in a year. One hundred years later the average Australian consumes 75 kilograms of sugar per annum!

This is a dramatic increase in a substance that isn't even a food and can cause the pancreas to overwork and our overall health to be negatively affected. A small taste of a delicious dessert can be as satisfying as wolfing down a whole bar of cheap chocolate.

By following a healthy way of eating you will find that such cravings will diminish. And by cooking or preparing the following sweet treats you can gradually educate yourself away from quick sugar fixes.

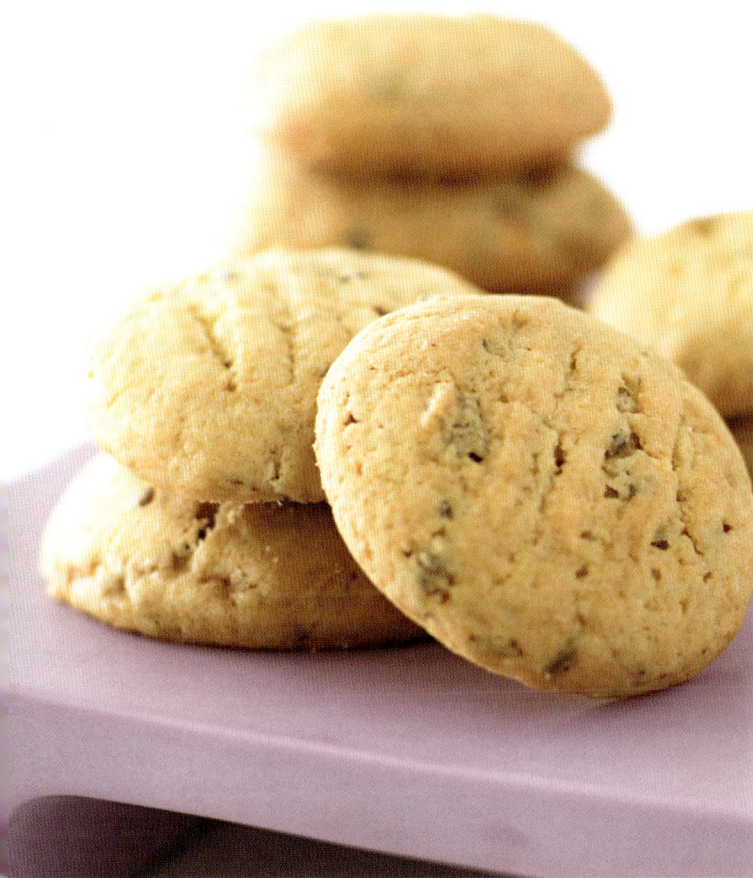
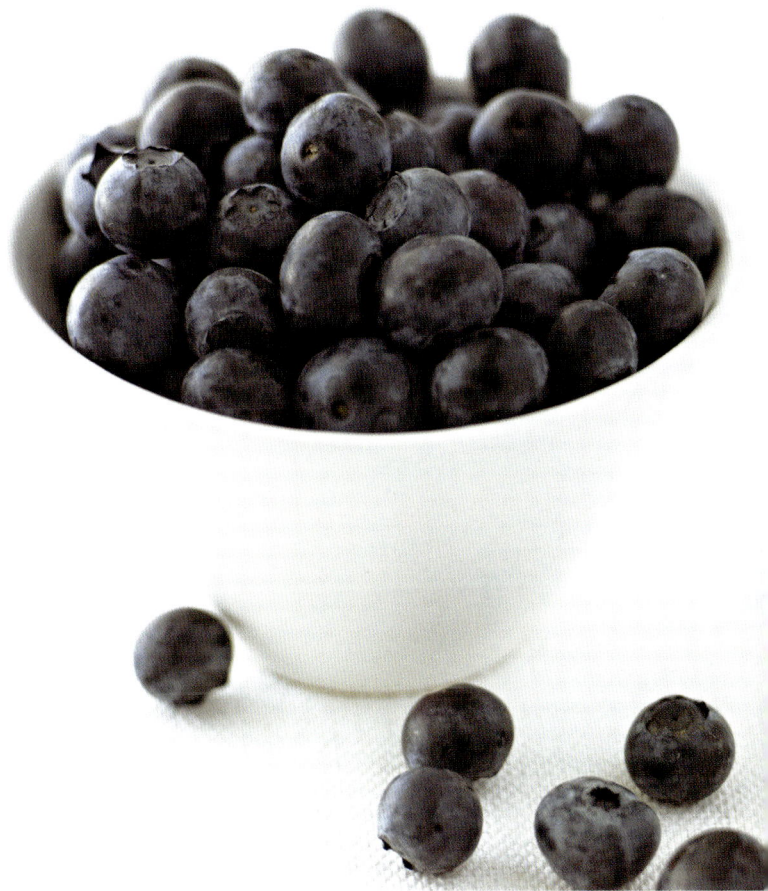

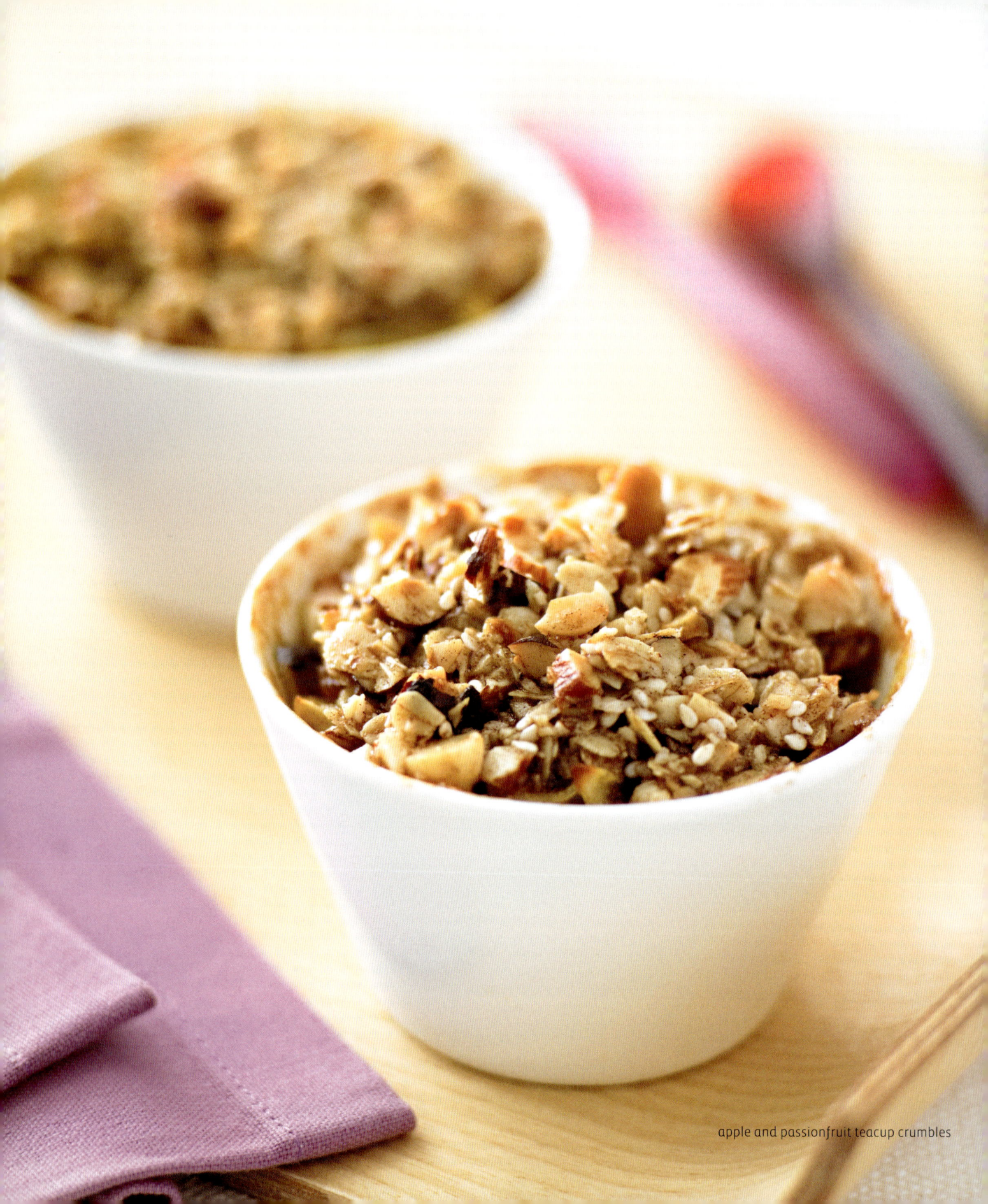

apple and passionfruit teacup crumbles

apple and passionfruit teacup crumbles

These fruity crumbles made in teacups or ramekins are irresistible. You can also make this in a baking dish. Apple concentrate is available in health food stores.

6 Granny Smith apples
1 cup apple concentrate
  or 2 tablespoons sugar in $1/4$ cup water
6 passionfruits, halved and flesh scooped out
$2/3$ cup nuts, roughly chopped
  (hazelnuts, almonds, macadamias etc.)
1 tablespoon sesame seeds
1 teaspoon cinnamon
75g butter, melted
$1/3$ cup maple syrup
$1/2$ cup rolled oats

Preheat the oven to 180°C. Peel, core and thinly slice the apples. Place apples in a saucepan with the apple concentrate. Cover and gently cook over low heat for 8–10 minutes or until soft. Stir through the passionfruit pulp and spoon into 6 teacups or ramekins.

Combine the chopped nuts, sesame seeds, cinnamon, melted butter, maple syrup and rolled oats. Sprinkle over the apple and passionfruit mixture in the teacups. Place on a baking tray and bake for 20 minutes or until golden and the crumble is cooked. Serves 6.

rhubarb crumble

It's hard to beat a fruit crumble on a chilly winter's evening. This one uses rhubarb, quince and pears. You can use green apples instead of the quinces if you prefer. The ground linseed, sunflower and almond meal (LSA) is available from health food shops.

8 sticks rhubarb, chopped into 6cm lengths
1 cup water
2 teaspoons orange zest
2 vanilla beans
3 cinnamon sticks
$1/4$ cup honey
2 large green pears, quartered and cored
1 large quince, scrubbed, cored and sliced
  or 2 green apples, cored and quartered
2 teaspoons ground nutmeg
1 tablespoon arrowroot

crumble
1 cup LSA (linseed, sunflower and almond meal)
1 cup shredded coconut
1 cup rolled oats
$1/2$ cup hazelnut meal
$1/2$ cup brown sugar
1 tablespoon buckwheat flour
2 tablespoons coconut oil or unsalted butter

Preheat over to 180°C. Lightly grease a deep baking dish.

Simmer rhubarb, water, orange zest, vanilla beans, cinnamon sticks and brown sugar or honey for about 10 minutes or until tender. Reserve syrup.

Then simmer the pears, quince (or apples) and nutmeg. This will take 10–15 minutes. Set aside, reserving the cooking liquid for a syrup topping and remove cinnamon sticks. Thicken the combined syrups with a tablespoon of arrowroot stirred in over a medium heat. Mix crumble ingredients together.

Mix together cooked fruits and arrange in a baking dish. Top with crumble mix and bake for 25–30 minutes or until golden brown. Serve with syrup and yoghurt. Serves 6.

baked fruit parcels

You can vary the fruit in these parcels according to what is in season. Defrosted berries can be used if fresh ones aren't available. Substitute the pears and apples with stone fruit when in season.

2 bananas, cut into chunks
2 pears, peeled and cut into wedges
1 apple, peeled and cut into wedges
1 punnet blueberries
pulp of 2–3 passionfruits
coconut cream to serve

Preheat the oven to 200ºC. Cut 4 lengths of baking paper (about 20cmx20cm) and place a quarter of each fruit in the centre of the 4 sheets.

Fold the baking paper around the fruit to form secure parcels and place on a baking tray. Bake in the oven for 15 minutes or until the fruit is hot and fragrant. Let each person open their own parcel and serve with coconut cream. Serves 4.

quince compote

We love to serve this as a winter dessert at the Centre. Many people don't know how to cook quinces and so have never experienced their delicate, fragrant flavour. You don't need to peel or core the quinces but you do need to scrub them in water to remove the soft down that covers them. Then use a sharp knife to cut them into wedges.

500ml water
2 tablespoons lemon juice
2 cups apple juice concentrate
1 cinnamon stick
2 star anise
1kg quince, scrubbed and cut into wedges

Bring the water to the boil in a medium saucepan. Add the lemon juice, apple juice concentrate, cinnamon and star anise. Bring to the boil and simmer for 5 minutes. Add the quince wedges and simmer until tender and the syrup turns pink. (The cooking time varies considerably so test to see whether the fruit is tender.) When it is cooked, remove with a slotted spoon and continue to cook the syrup until reduced by about half and a reddish-pink. Pour the syrup over the cooked quince. Serve warm or cold. Serves 4.

citrus stacks with berries

Defrosted berries can be used in this recipe if fresh ones aren't available.

2 oranges
2 blood oranges
4 tablespoons maple syrup (optional)
1 cup mixed berries

Using a small serrated knife, cut the peel and pith off the oranges and blood oranges. (Do this over a bowl to catch the juices.) Cut the oranges into 1cm slices and assemble on plates, alternating the orange with blood orange. Pour over any collected juice and maple syrup (if using). Scatter with berries. Serves 4.

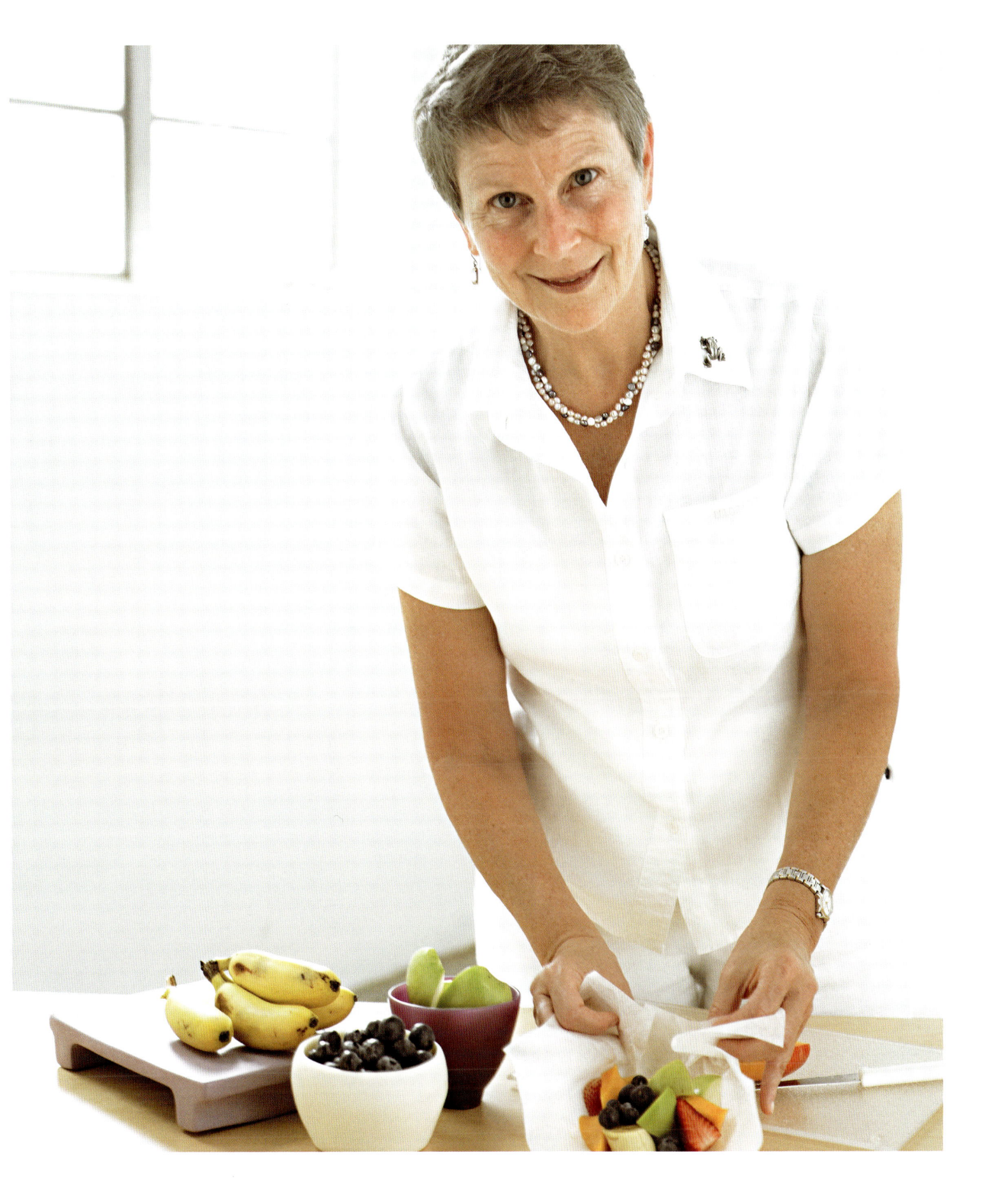

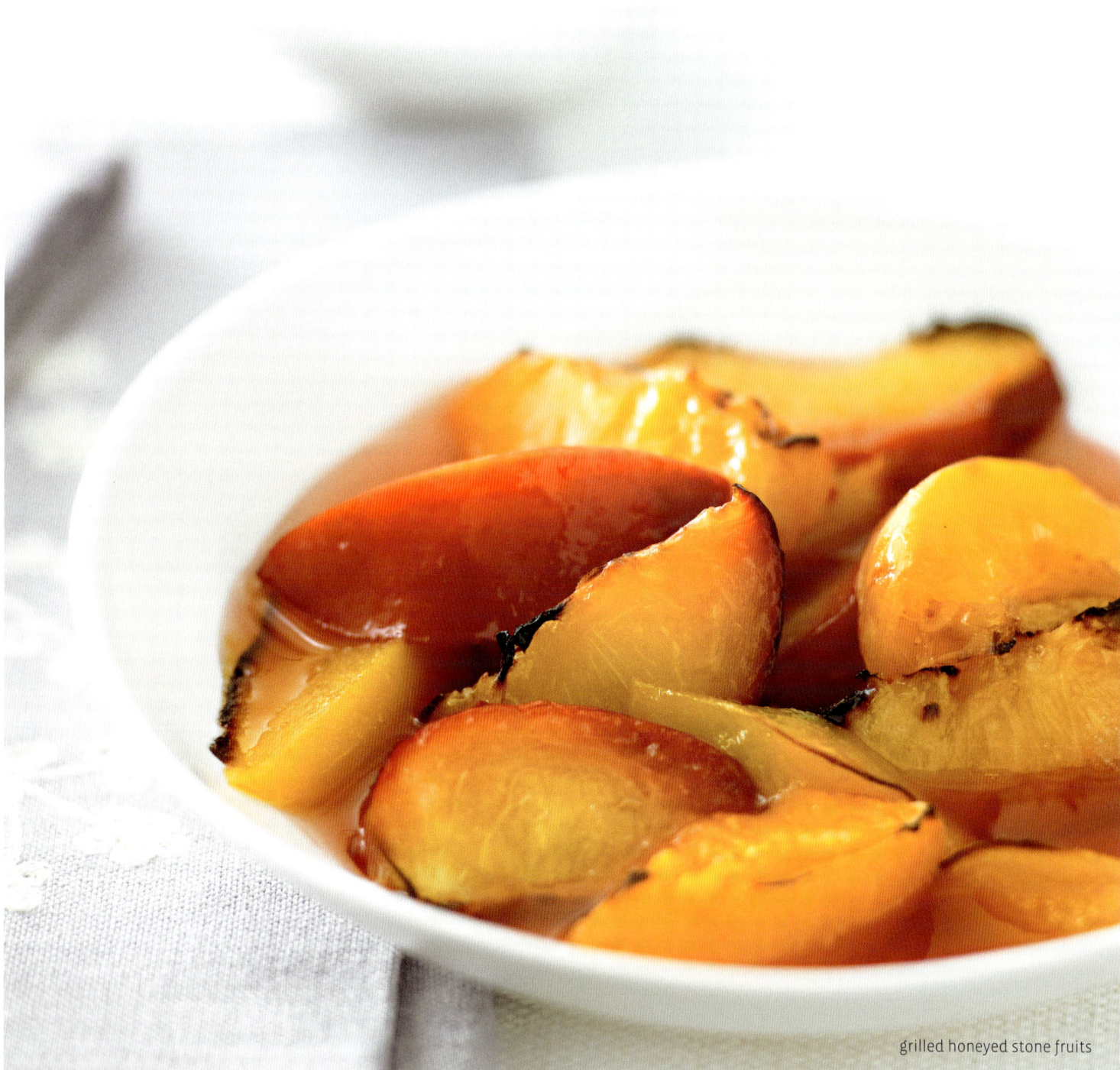

grilled honeyed stone fruits

roast pineapple wedges with shaved coconut

The best way to pick a ripe pineapple is by pulling a leaf from its crown. It should come away easily. Pineapples don't ripen after being picked so it's best to eat them soon after purchase. Pineapples are packed with vitamin C, a digestive enzyme called bromelain and loads of fibre.

$1/3$ cup shaved dried coconut
1 medium pineapple
$1/2$ cup raw sugar
2 teaspoons grated lime zest
1–2 tablespoons lime juice

Preheat the oven to 180°C. Place the shaved coconut on a baking tray and bake for 8 minutes or until golden.

Turn on the grill and line a tray with foil. Peel the pineapple and cut lengthways into 12 wedges. Combine the sugar and zest and lightly coat the wedges with the mixture. Place on the grill tray and grill for about 8 minutes or until caramelised and warm.

Drizzle with the lime juice and scatter with the roasted coconut shavings. Serves 6.

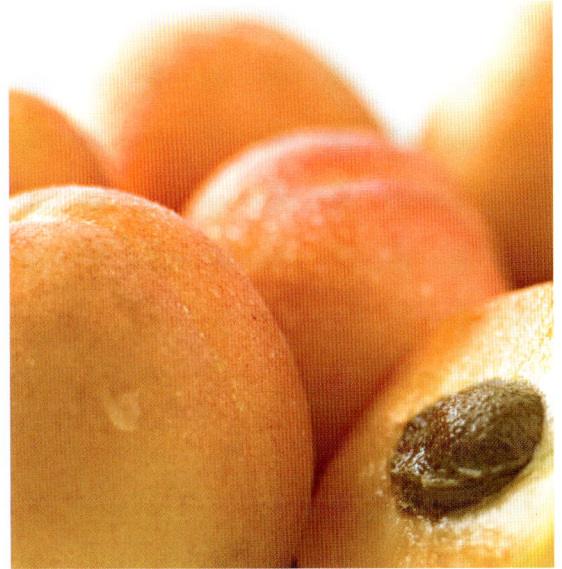

grilled honeyed stone fruits

Simple and luscious when using perfectly ripe fruit, this dessert couldn't be more delicious.

4 plums
3 nectarines
2 mangoes
4 fresh apricots
$1/4$ cup warm honey
plain yoghurt to serve

Thoroughly wash the fruit, remove the stones and pips and cut into thick wedges. Place in a single layer in a large baking dish. Drizzle with the honey.

Preheat the grill, place the baking dish under the grill and cook the fruit for 4–5 minutes or until heated and golden. Serve immediately with a spoonful of yoghurt. Serves 4.

Freshly made fruit salads provide an abundance of vitamins, antioxidants and nutrients to cleanse, nourish and rejuvenate our bodies.

tropical fruit salad

You can vary this beautiful concoction with different tropical fruits. Palm sugar is found in Asian supermarkets or you can use soft brown sugar or raw sugar instead.

$1/3$ cup grated palm sugar
$1/4$ cup water
2 limes, juiced
2 ripe mangoes, peeled, seeded and chopped
12 fresh lychees or 12 rambutans, peeled and pitted
$1/2$ small pineapple, peeled and chopped
2 small bananas

Place the sugar and water in a small saucepan and gently heat until the sugar dissolves. Bring to the boil, then reduce the heat and simmer for 2 minutes. Remove from the heat and cool. Add the lime juice.

Arrange the fruit on a deep platter and pour over the syrup. Serves 6.

pawpaw and melon salad

A delectable summer dessert always making the most of the season's fruits.

$1^{1}/2$ cups water
$1/2$ cup honey
$1^{1}/2$ tablespoons ginger, shredded
$1/2$ cup mint leaves, shredded
2 tablespoons lime juice
$1/2$ honeydew melon
$1/2$ rockmelon
large wedge seedless watermelon
$1/2$ pawpaw
shredded mint leaves to serve

To make the syrup, place water, honey, ginger, mint leaves and lime juice in a saucepan. Bring to the boil while stirring to dissolve the honey. Reduce the heat and simmer for 10 minutes. Allow to cool and chill in fridge.

Peel and seed the melons and pawpaw. Cut into thick wedges and place on a serving plate. Pour syrup through a sieve to remove shredded ginger and mint. Spoon over the chilled syrup and scatter with shredded mint leaves. Serves 4.

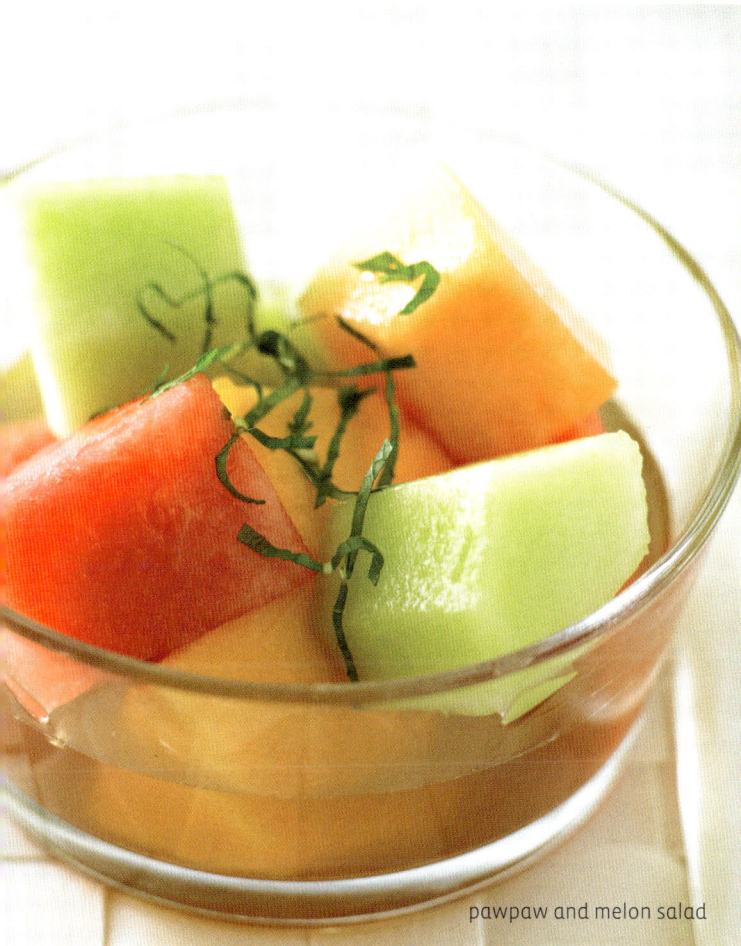

pawpaw and melon salad

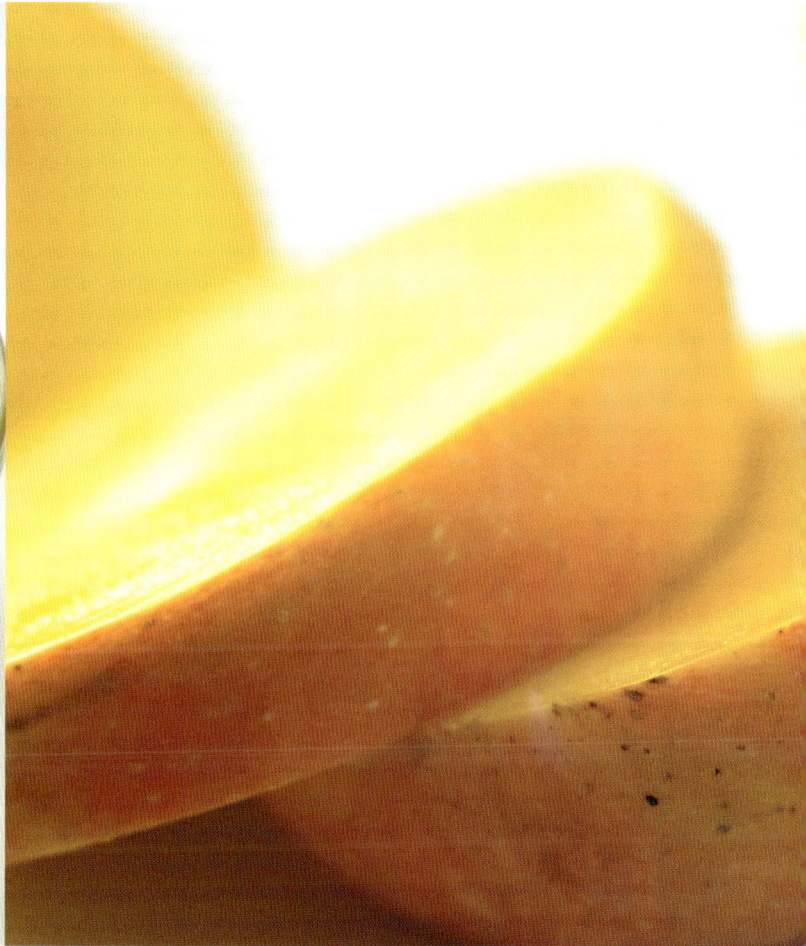

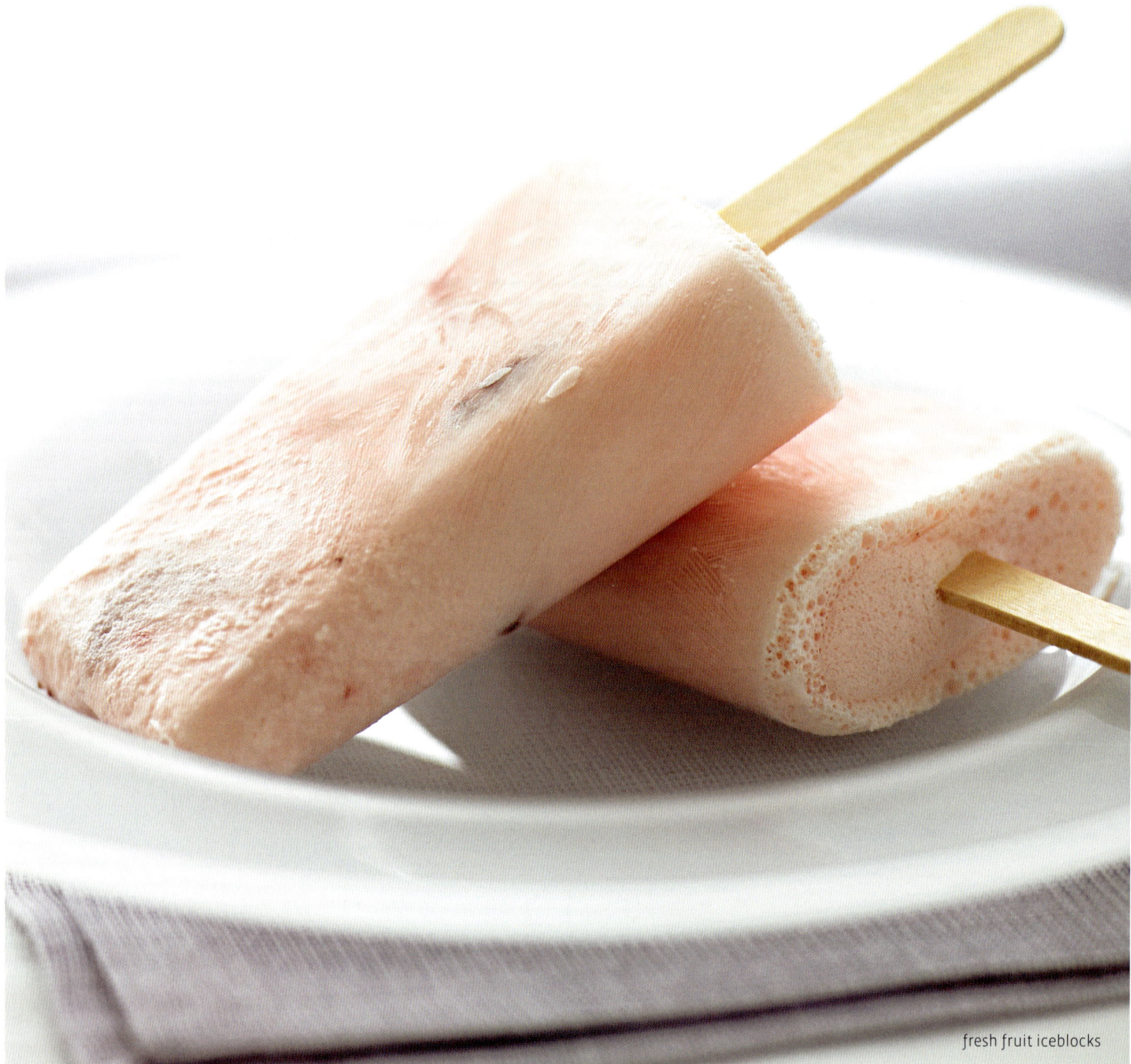

fresh fruit iceblocks

bliss bombs

These bliss bombs satisfy a sweet craving and are nutritious at the same time. They can be kept in the fridge for a few days if you can resist eating them! Carob powder is available in health food stores and 70 or 85 per cent Lindt chocolate is readily available.

bliss bombs

8 tablespoons carob powder
8 tablespoons tahini, preferably from unhulled sesame seeds
4 tablespoons honey
1 tablespoon sunflower seeds
1 tablespoon pepitas, soaked, rinsed and drained
2 tablespoons coconut cream (optional)

coating

$1/2$ cup dark Lindt chocolate, grated
$1/4$ cup sesame seeds, soaked, rinsed and drained or $1/2$ cup desiccated coconut

Mix the carob powder, tahini, honey, sunflower seeds, pepitas and coconut cream (if using) until they form a dough-like mixture. Adjust consistency by making more moist with tahini or honey or drier with more carob. Roll the mixture into balls and coat with either the chocolate and sesame seed combination or chocolate and coconut. Makes 12–15 bliss bombs.

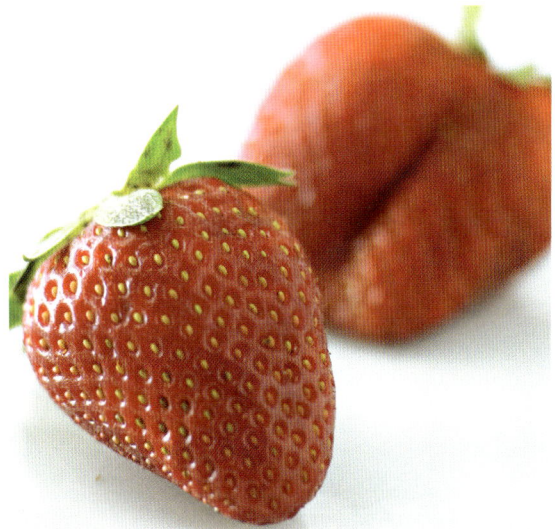

fresh fruit iceblocks

These are so refreshing on a hot summer's day, and they're packed with goodness without any artificial flavours or colours. For a change, you can use other fruits instead of strawberries, and coconut milk instead of the yoghurt.

250g strawberries, roughly chopped
2 cups plain yoghurt
$3/4$ cup apple juice
$1/4$ cup apple concentrate
1 tablespoon lemon juice

Place half the chopped strawberries in a food processor or blender. Add the yoghurt, apple juice, apple concentrate and lemon juice and blend until well combined. Fold through the remaining strawberries.

Pour mixture into iceblock moulds, cover with the tops and freeze for 3–4 hours or until frozen. If using moulds with wooden sticks, freeze the mixture until it's frozen enough to support the wooden sticks (about 40 minutes) then place wooden sticks in the centre of the iceblocks.

Put back in the freezer until frozen. Remove fruit iceblocks from moulds to serve. Makes 10 iceblocks.

lemon and passionfruit delicious

This is one of those miraculous dishes in which you transform a bowl of unassuming ingredients into a lovely dessert with soft cake on top and a tangy sauce beneath.

1/2 cup raw sugar
1/4 cup plain flour, sifted
zest of 1 lemon
1/4 cup lemon juice
pulp of 3 passionfruits
50g butter, melted
3 eggs, separated
1 1/2 cups milk (cow, oat, brown rice or coconut)

Preheat the oven to 180°C. Place the sugar, flour, lemon zest and juice, passionfruit, melted butter and egg yolks in a large mixing bowl and beat until well combined. Add the milk to the mixture and combine well.

Whisk the egg whites until stiff. Fold into the lemon and passionfruit mixture. Pour into an ovenproof dish and bake in the oven for 30 minutes or until the top of the pudding is golden and cooked.

Serve warm with plain yoghurt or coconut cream. Serves 4.

chocolate and hazelnut cake

Every cookbook needs a chocolate cake recipe and this one is no exception. Use the 85 per cent Lindt chocolate if possible. The zucchini gives a delicious moist texture to the cake.

300g dark Lindt chocolate, chopped
200g unsalted butter
5 eggs, separated
1 cup raw or brown sugar
1 teaspoon vanilla extract
2 cups of hazelnuts, whizzed in a food processor until fine
1 cup zucchini, grated
1 cup wholemeal flour
1 teaspoon baking powder
chopped hazelnuts, grated chocolate and orange to serve

Preheat the oven to 160°C. Brush a 22cm round cake tin with melted butter or coconut oil. Line the base with baking paper.

Gently melt the chocolate and butter in a saucepan stirring until smooth. Using electric beaters, whisk the egg whites until stiff.

Place the egg yolks, sugar and vanilla in a medium-size bowl and using the electric beaters (no need to wash from whisking the egg whites), whisk until creamy. Fold the hazelnuts and zucchini through the chocolate mixture until well combined. Fold in the flour and baking powder, then using a metal spoon, fold through the stiffened egg whites and pour into the prepared cake tin. Bake for 1 1/4 hours or until a skewer inserted into the centre of the cake comes out clean.

Cool in the tin for 20 minutes then turn out onto a wire rack to cool. Decorate with chopped hazelnuts and grated chocolate. Serve with segments of fresh orange.

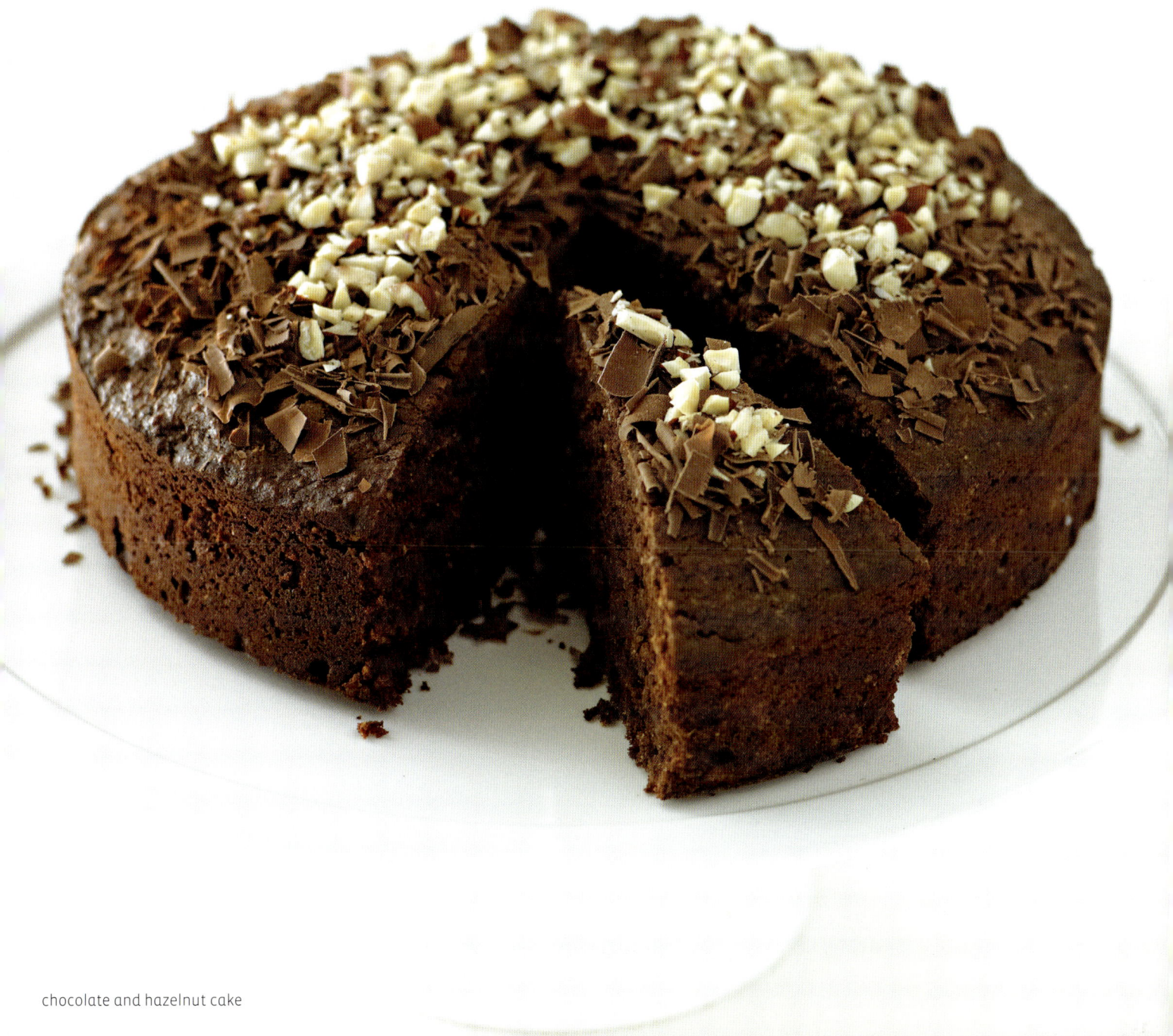

chocolate and hazelnut cake

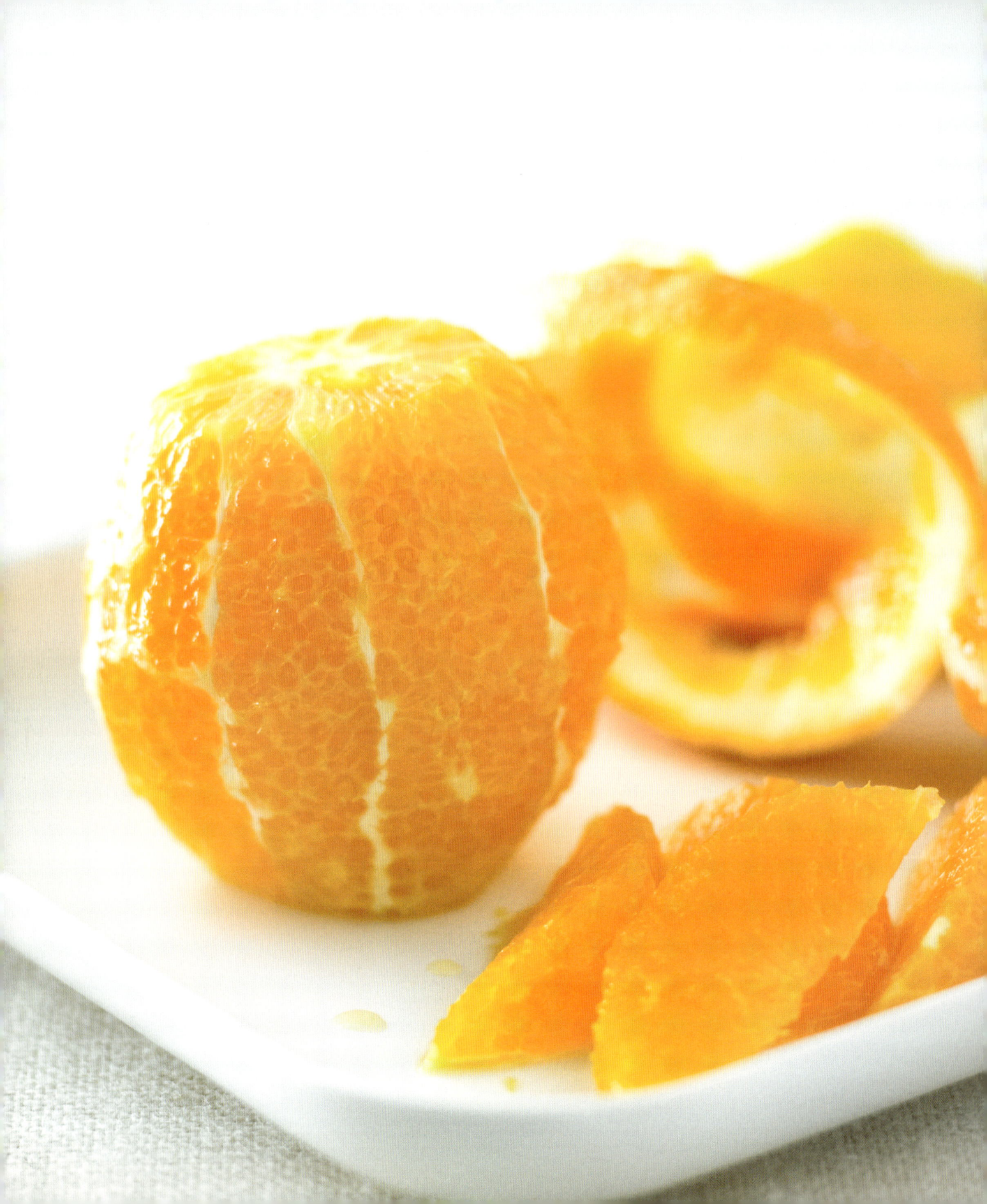

orange and lemon polenta cake

4 eggs, separated
1/3 cup raw sugar
2 teaspoons orange zest
2 teaspoons lemon zest
1/2 cup orange juice
1/2 cup polenta
2/3 cup self-raising flour
1/3 cup pistachio kernels, whizzed in food processor

syrup
1 cup honey
1/2 cup orange juice
1 tablespoon orange zest
5 fresh figs, cut into wedges

Preheat oven to 180ºC. Lightly grease a 22cm cake tin.

Whisk egg yolks, sugar and orange and lemon zest and stir in juice and polenta. Add in flour and pistachios. Whisk the egg whites until stiff and fold into the polenta mixture and pour into cake tin. Bake for 30 minutes or until a skewer inserted into the middle comes out clean.

Make a syrup by heating together the honey, orange juice and zest in a saucepan over a moderate heat. Pour half of the syrup over the cake on the wire rack. Place figs in the remaining syrup and set aside to cool. Top each slice of cake with a fig segment and drizzle over syrup.

orange and almond cake

For those who can't eat gluten this is the cake for you — moist and full of Mediterranean flavour. It's also remarkably easy to make and only requires 6 ingredients!

2 oranges
6 eggs
1 1/2 cups almond meal (ground almonds)
1/2 cup raw sugar
1 teaspoon baking powder
icing sugar to serve

Place the whole oranges in a saucepan and cover with water. Bring to the boil then reduce the heat and simmer for 45 minutes or until tender. Remove from the water and cool.

Preheat the oven to 180ºC. Lightly grease a 22cm round cake tin and line the base with baking paper. Cut each orange into quarters and remove any pips. Place the orange quarters (yes, including the skins!) into a blender or food processor and blend until smooth.

Place the eggs in a mixing bowl and lightly beat. Fold through the orange puree, almond meal, sugar and baking powder. Pour the mixture into the prepared tin. Bake for 45–50 minutes or until firm. Leave to cool in the tin. Serve lightly dusted with icing sugar.

carrot cake

There is plenty of good nutrition in this popular recipe and it will never last long!

1 cup self-raising flour
1 teaspoon baking powder
1 cup wholemeal plain flour
1 teaspoon ground cinnamon
1 teaspoon ground mixed spice
1 teaspoon ground nutmeg
$^1/_2$ cup LSA (linseed, sunflower and almond meal)
$^1/_2$ cup chopped walnuts
$^1/_2$ cup shredded coconut
2 teaspoons lemon zest
4 eggs, separated
1 teaspoon vanilla essence
$^1/_2$ cup golden syrup
$^1/_2$ cup brown sugar
$^1/_2$ cup coconut milk
80mls coconut or extra-virgin olive oil
2 cups carrot, grated and sautéed in extra-virgin olive
 or coconut oil
plain yoghurt, cinnamon and maple syrup to serve

Preset over to 180ºC. Lightly grease and line a 22cm round cake tin.

Whisk egg whites until stiff. In a large bowl sift together the flours and spices. Add LSA, walnuts and coconut and lightly mix through. In a separate bowl, using a food processor, electric beaters or whisk, combine the egg yolks, golden syrup, sugar, vanilla essence, lemon zest, coconut milk and oil.

Fold egg yolk mixture and sautéed carrot into the flour mixture and mix gently and well. Gently fold stiffened egg whites into the mixture and pour into a cake tin. Bake for 45 minutes or until skewer comes out clean.

Serve with yoghurt flavoured with cinnamon and a little maple syrup.

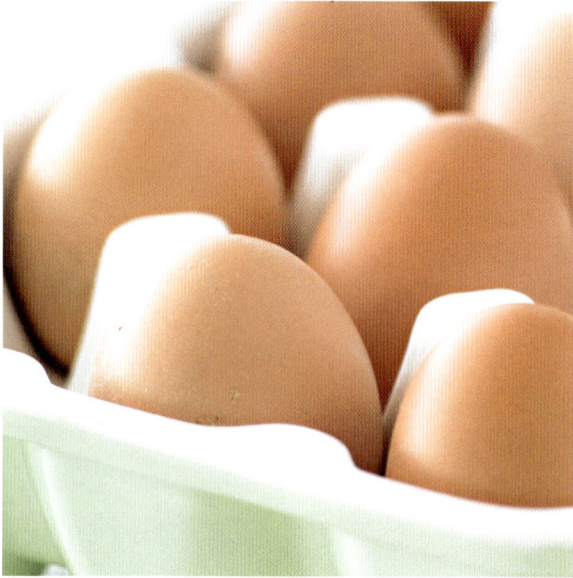

banana muffins

1 cup wholemeal self-raising flour
1 cup self-raising flour
$^1/_2$ cup brown or raw sugar
1 teaspoon finely grated lemon zest
1 teaspoon ground cinnamon
pinch ground cardamom
1 egg
1 cup buttermilk or coconut milk
2 tablespoons extra-virgin olive or coconut oil
1 cup ripe mashed banana

Preheat the oven to 180ºC. Lightly coat a 12-hole muffin tin with oil. Combine the flour, sugar, lemon zest, cinnamon and cardamom in a bowl.

Place the egg, milk, oil and mashed banana in another bowl and beat together with a fork. Fold into the flour mixture until just combined. Spoon evenly into the prepared tin. (If you like higher muffins, only fill a 10-muffin tin.)

Bake in the oven for 20–30 minutes or until cooked. (They should spring back when lightly pressed.) Remove from the tin and cool on a wire rack. Makes 12 muffins.

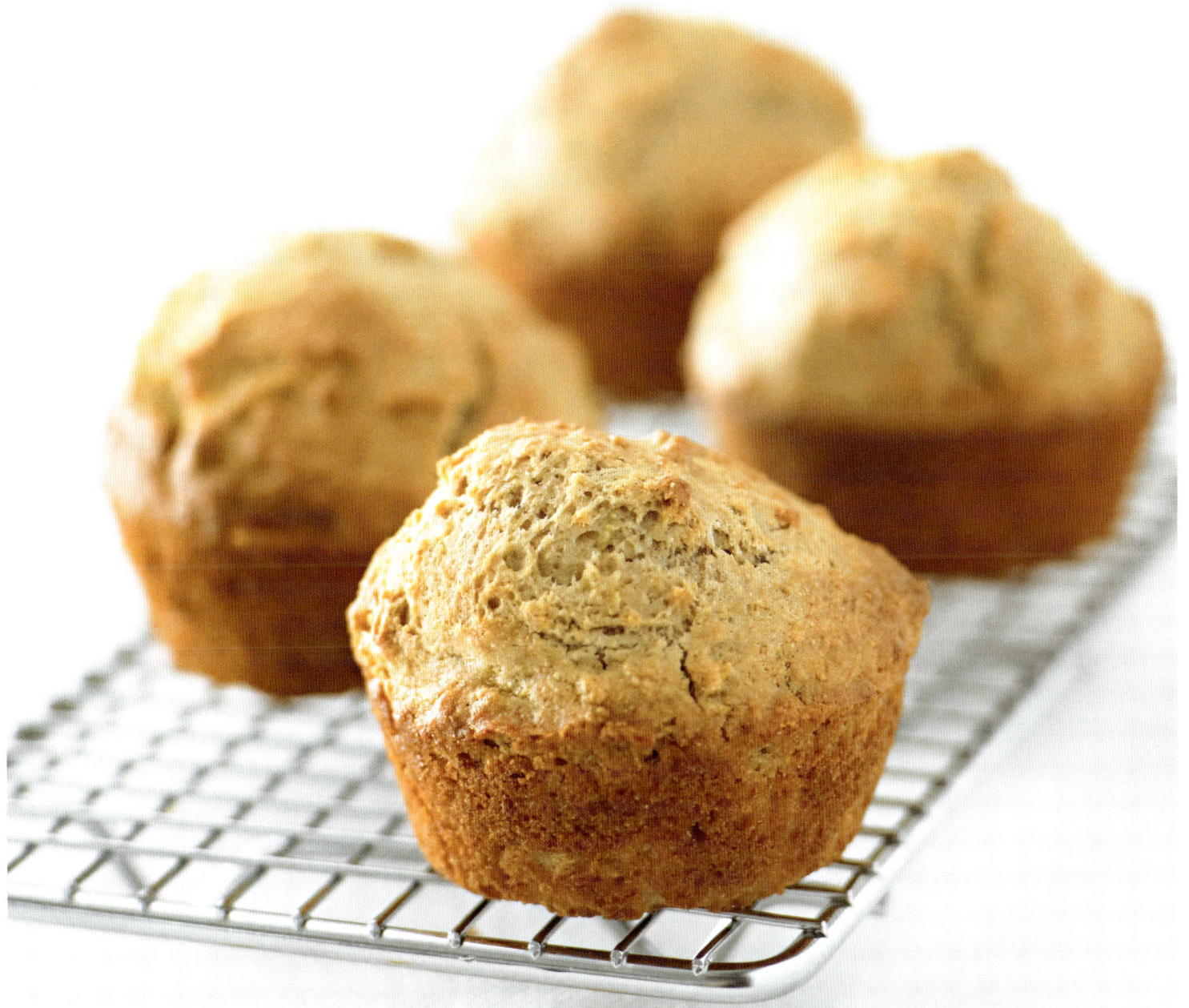

banana muffins

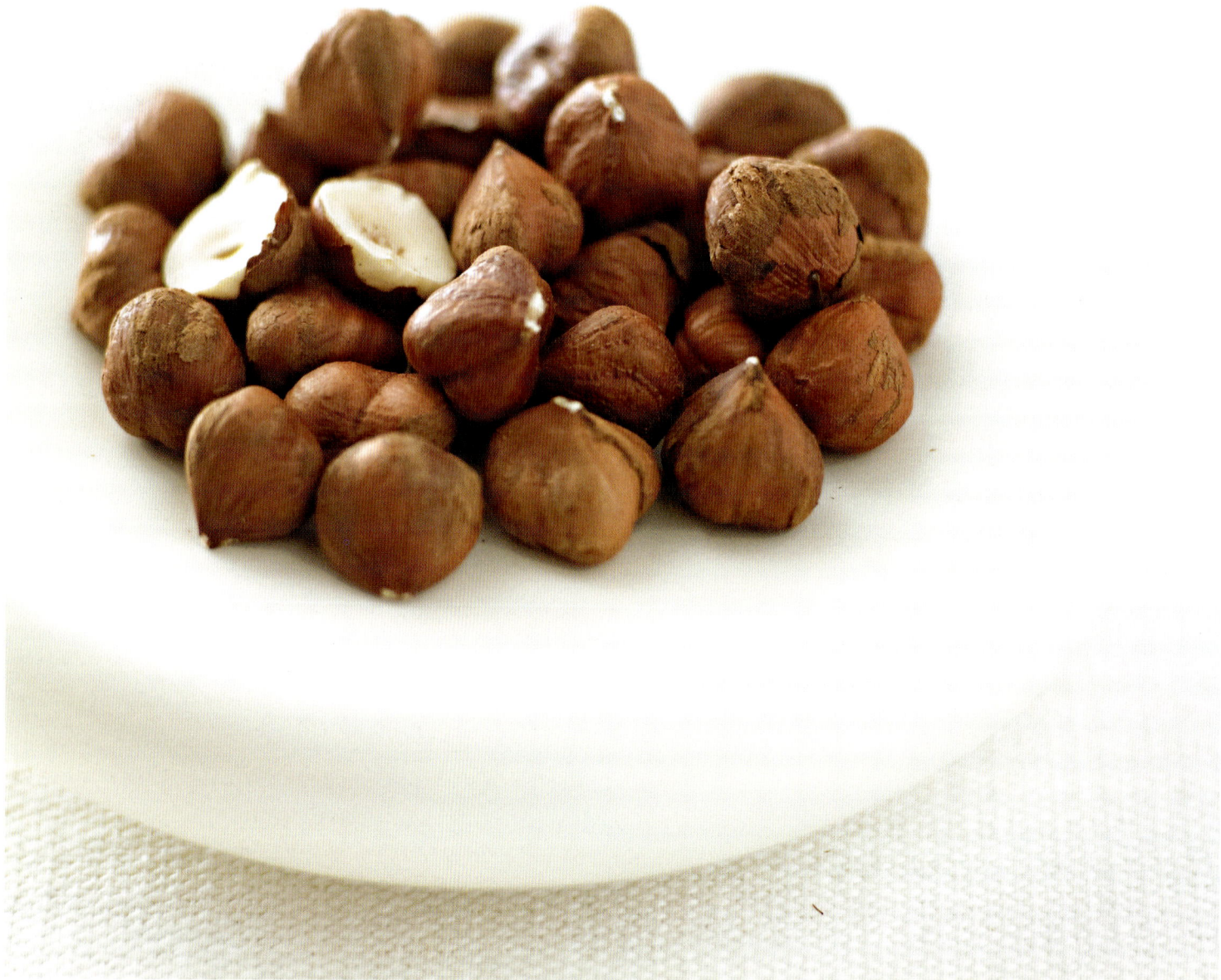

hazelnut and fig torte

200g hazelnuts
200g dried figs
1 cup water
100g dark chocolate, chopped (optional)
4 egg whites
1/2 cup raw sugar

Preheat the oven to 180°C and lightly grease an 18cm square cake tin, lining the base with baking paper. Place the hazelnuts on a baking tray and roast for 10 minutes. Place the figs in a saucepan with the water and bring to the boil. Reduce the heat and simmer for 10 minutes, then drain and blend in a food processor until smooth.

Place the hazelnuts in a clean tea towel and rub off the skins and cool. When completely cool, place in a food processor along with the chocolate (if using), and blend until coarse crumbs.

Beat the egg whites in a large bowl until soft peaks form. Add the sugar gradually while continuing to beat. Fold through the hazelnut mixture and then the fig puree. Pour the mixture into the prepared tin. Bake for 35–40 minutes or until the torte starts to come away from the sides of the tin. Leave to cool in the tin. To serve, cut into squares and drizzle with yoghurt or serve with coconut cream.

SUGAR

Aim for no more than two dessertspoons of added sugar per day with a maximum of four dessertspoons occasionally. We live in a very sugar-oriented society and many of us have a pronounced sweet tooth. Excess sugar is responsible for all kinds of health problems including obesity which can lead to high blood pressure, type 2 diabetes and a compromised immune system.

Try to reduce all artificial sweeteners — they might please the tongue but are a source of chemicals your body was never designed to process. Apple juice concentrate and dried fruits are better sugar substitutes in dishes that require some sweetening. Xylitol is a natural sugar substitute derived from birch trees and can be used as a sugar substitute in any of the recipes. It is readily available in health food stores.

date scones

These scones are delicious for afternoon tea. The dates provide fibre, flavour and a natural sweetness that makes them irresistible.

125g unsalted butter
4 cups self-raising flour
2 eggs, lightly beaten
1/2 cup milk (cow or oat)
3/4 cup pitted dried dates, roughly chopped

Preheat the oven to 220°C. Place butter and flour in a food processor and pulse until well combined. Add the dates and pulse. Add the eggs and milk and briefly pulse again. Tip the mixture onto a clean workbench, sprinkled with a little flour, and quickly knead into a smooth dough. Don't overwork the mixture.

Roll or press out into a 1.5cm deep dish. Using a round cutter, cut the dough into scones. Place on a baking tray and cook in the oven for 12–15 minutes or until golden. Delicious served warm with jam, but great at room temperature too. Makes about 20 scones.

oat crunchies

These delicious morsels are full of healthy fibre and natural ingredients.

4 Weetbix, well crushed
1 cup rolled oats
1 tablespoon sesame seeds, toasted in a small frying pan
1/2 cup desiccated coconut
1/2 cup soft brown sugar
1 teaspoon ground cinnamon (optional)
1 teaspoon ground allspice (optional)
125g unsalted butter, melted
1 tablespoon honey

Preheat oven to 180°C and line a 25cmx16cm (or thereabouts) slice pan with a sheet of baking paper, overlapping 2 sides. (It's fine to leave the other 2 sides not lined.)

Combine the crushed Weetbix, oats, sesame seeds, coconut, sugar, cinnamon and spice (if using) in a mixing bowl. Stir through the melted butter and honey and combine well. Spoon the mixture into the prepared pan and flatten down.

Bake in the oven for 15 minutes or until golden brown. Remove from the oven and allow to cool. Cut into small squares and store in an airtight container.

rosemary or lavender biscuits

These aromatic biscuits are a special treat for our guests to accompany morning tea or coffee. Choose whether you prefer to use rosemary or lavender — both are lovely. They can also be frozen after cooking.

125g unsalted butter, softened
1/3 cup soft brown or raw sugar
1 egg
3/4 cup self-raising flour, sifted
1/2 cup plain flour, sifted
2 teaspoons custard powder
1–2 teaspoons fresh rosemary leaves, finely chopped or 1–2 teaspoons dried English lavender (check that there are no additives), removed from stem and chopped

Place butter and sugar in a food processor and blend until creamy. Add the egg and pulse until combined. Add the self-raising and plain flours and custard powder and rosemary or lavender and pulse until combined. Place in the fridge for 30 minutes.

Preheat the oven to 200°C. Form the mixture into small balls (about 2 teaspoons of mixture), and place on a baking tray lined with baking paper. Press down with a fork to form a biscuit and bake for 12–15 minutes or until golden.

Leave to cool on the baking tray—if you can resist eating them warm—and then store in an airtight container or freeze for later.

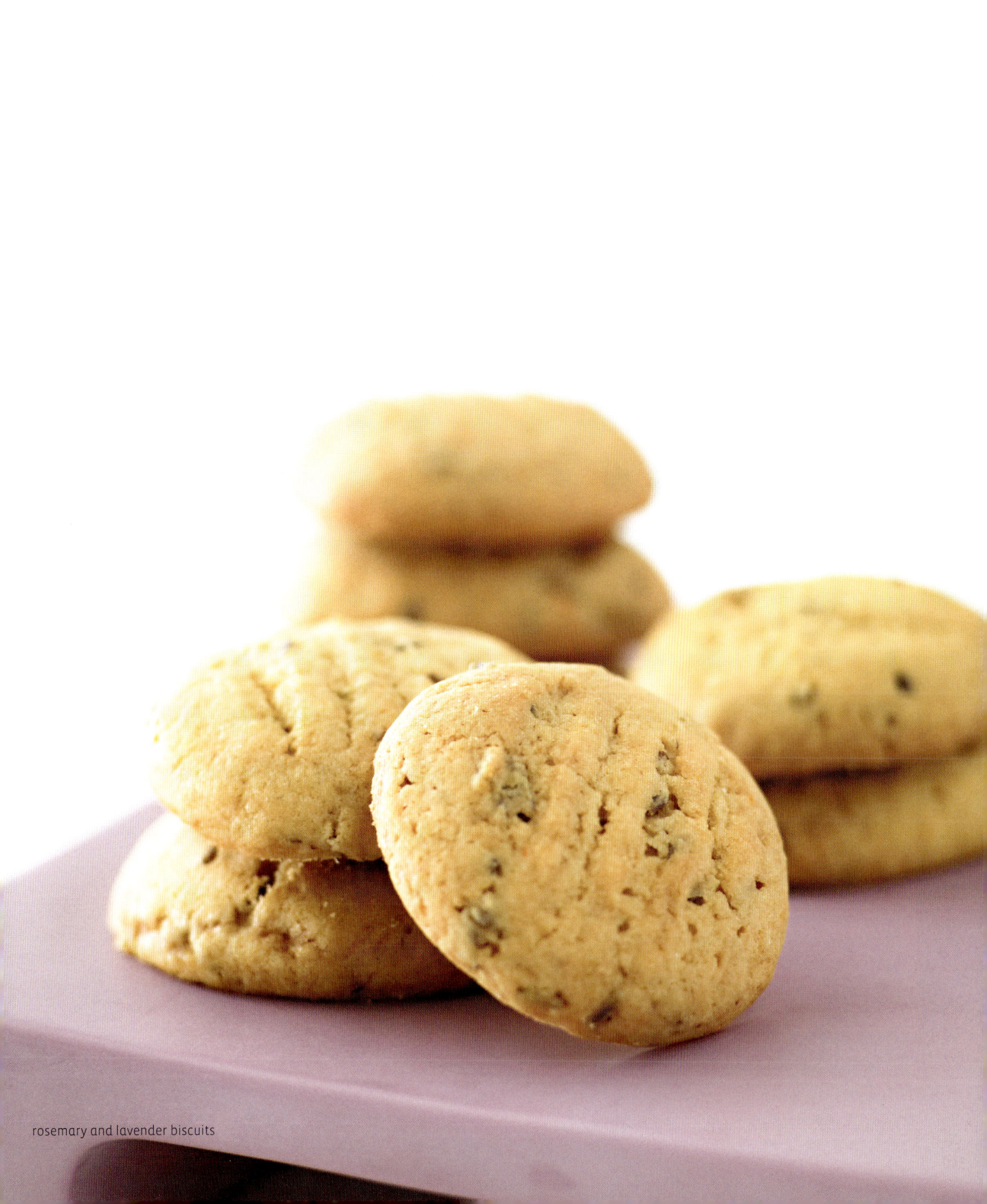

rosemary and lavender biscuits

The Petrea King Quest for Life Centre

At the Petrea King Quest for Life Centre, we give people practical strategies for living well in challenging circumstances and for finding meaning in the midst of life's unexpected events.

WE RECOGNISE THAT we can't always change what happens to us in life but we can play an active role in how we're going to respond to what happens to us. We value peace of mind above all else.

There are many events in life that stop us in our tracks and cause us to consider how best to meet the challenge we face: an unexpected diagnosis, an accident, loss or tragedy can be such an impetus.

Some people seek more meaningful ways of managing the challenging circumstances of chronic illness, multiple loss, anxiety, relationship breakdown, depression or the consequences of past abuse. Other people choose to take time out to review their life with the intention of deepening their relationship with themselves and living a more satisfying and meaningful life.

Since 1985 more than 60,000 people have attended residential programs or counselling with Petrea and her team of trained health professionals.

Since 1999 our residential programs and services have been conducted at the Quest for Life Centre — an historic guesthouse set in 3.6 tranquil hectares of gardens at Bundanoon, in the beautiful Southern Highlands of New South Wales.

If you feel we can assist you through one of our residential programs or other services, please call us with your particular needs. We look forward to our paths crossing with yours.

The Quest for Life Foundation

The Petrea King Quest for Life Centre is owned and operated by the Quest for Life Foundation, a registered charity established in 1990 by Petrea King. Proceeds from the sale of this book go to support the work of the Quest for Life Foundation.

The Quest for Life Foundation subsidises all programs as well as an additional subsidy with the support of the NSW Health Department for people on pensions and low incomes.

Donations assist us to support the provision and expansion of our services and are fully tax deductible.

Petrea King Quest for Life Centre
PO Box 390
Bundanoon NSW 2578
Australia

Ph: (61 2) 4883 6599
Fax: (61 2) 4883 6755
E-mail: info@questforlife.com.au
Web: www.questforlife.com.au